600 MCQs in Anaesthesia: Basic Sciences

P. J. Simpson
MD FFARCS
Consultant Anaesthetist,
Frenchay Hospital, Bristol;
Senior Clinical Lecturer,
University of Bristol

N. W. Goodman
MA DPhil BM BCh FFARCS
Lecturer in Anaesthesia,
University of Bristol

Churchill Livingstone

EDINBURGH LONDON MELBOURNE AND NEW YORK 1985

CHURCHILL LIVINGSTONE
Medical Division of Longman Group UK Limited

Distributed in the United States of America by
Churchill Livingstone Inc., 1560 Broadway, New York,
N.Y. 10036, and by associated companies, branches
and representatives throughout the world.

First published 1985
  Reprinted 1988
  Reprinted 1989

ISBN 0 443 03041 3

British Library Cataloguing in Publication Data
  Simpson, Peter J.
  600 MCQs in anaesthesia: basic sciences.
  1. Anesthesia—Problems, exercises, etc,
  I. Title II. Goodman, N. W.
  617'.96'076 RD82.3

Library of Congress Cataloging in Publication Data
Simpson, P.J.
  600 MCQs in anaesthesia; basic sciences
  Includes index.
  1. Anesthesiology—Examinations, questions, etc.
2. Medical sciences—Examinations, questions, etc.
I. Simpson, Peter J. II. Title. III. Title: Six
hundred multiple choice questions on the basic sciences
for the FFARCS. [DNLM: 1. Anesthesiology—examination
questions. 2. Science—examination questions.
WO 218 G653z]
RD82.3.G66 1985 617'.96'076 84–23072

Produced by Longman Group (FE) Limited
Printed in Hong Kong

Preface

This book aims to provide examination practice at Multiple Choice Questions on the Basic Sciences for the diploma of FFARCS. The questions are arranged in mock papers of 60 MCQs (20 Physiology, 20 Pharmacology, 20 Physics, followed by the answers) to allow candidates to time themselves answering questions similar to those likely to be encountered in the actual examination. It will help with the need to get a "feel" for MCQ "technique" before turning to the "real thing" in the examination hall.

Unlike those books of MCQs arranged under topic headings, candidates will have to be adaptable, not only to changing topic from question to question, but also to the degree of difficulty — and, as is bound to happen in the actual examination, candidates will find that there are some questions which they cannot answer.

The compilation of the papers has been greatly eased by the use of a PDP-11 computer on which all the questions were stored, edited, sorted into subject headings and finally cross-checked to avoid duplication and to provide a balance within each paper.

The questions have evolved over a number of years of organising courses and providing MCQ question practice for the FFARCS and we must acknowledge the help of colleagues and candidates past and present in the Nuffield Department of Anaesthetics, Oxford and in the three Teaching Hospitals in Bristol: Frenchay, Southmead and Bristol Royal Infirmary.

1985

P. J. Simpson
N. W. Goodman

Introduction

There are two things that you must do to pass the examinations for the diploma of the FFARCS: you must reach a certain level of knowledge; and you must know how to present it to the examiners. This is the first of two books that are more concerned with the second of these requirements; they will also help you to assess your level of knowledge, but they should not be treated as sources of knowledge.

The standard textbooks are the best source books of basic knowledge for the FFARCS. The more specialised texts, reviews in the journals, and discussion with others should be used to build upon this knowledge — to update it, and to find faults in it. You cannot expect to pass an exam unless you work for it: the more clinically oriented is the exam, then the more importance you must place on gaining wide experience in clinical anaesthesia. You must avoid the danger of working too much "at the books."

Many people think that the key to these exams is to go on a course, and there is no doubt that courses can be extremely useful. They should, however, be thought of as a means of aiming one's studies in the right directions; it is disappointing to find that many people will attend a course 2-3 months before the hurdle of a major examination apparently without having done any work. This is foolhardy. To get the most out of a course, one should have covered some of the groundwork beforehand. Once you have acquired what you hope to be sufficient knowledge (and in the absence of a published syllabus this must sometimes be a matter of guesswork in some areas), then is the time that these books should be of help to you.

How to Answer Multiple Choice Questions

The format of the MCQs in the FFA examination is a stem and five branches. The stem may be short ("Opiates are:"), or may be a few lines, for example when presenting a clinical problem. Each of the five branches that follow may be true or false. You score one mark for each correct answer, minus one for each incorrect answer, and, extremely important to the exam technique, you score nothing if you choose not to answer a particular branch. Your actual answers are marked by computer, and so you must eventually put your answers onto special cards that are supplied separately. These cards have the question numbers printed on them and you indicate your answer by filling in a "true" or a "false" box in pencil.

The most important tactic is not to guess: if you don't know — leave that branch blank. You should also think very carefully if you think a branch (or a stem) is ambiguous.

You must read each stem very carefully: watch out for qualifying words such as "commonly", "rarely", "always" and the like because they can turn what would otherwise be a "false" into a "true" and vice versa. Re-read the stem with each statement: it is all too easy to forget the emphasis and exact wording of the stem as you work down the five branches. Watch out for negatives: in the heat of the moment you may fail to see "not" in a branch. "May" is an awkward word; one can argue that anything "may" cause anything else. Try to give the answer relevant to clinical practice: for instance, it is "true" that atropine may cause bradycardia, but not that propranolol may relieve bronchospasm.

There are some subjects on which questions tend to be particularly confusing: the oxyhaemoglobin dissociation curve is one, the ionic dissociation of drugs is another. These are both subjects in which the wording of stem and branch are crucial. If an option states, "The saturated vapour pressure of halothane is 243 mm Hg", then the answer is clear (if you happen to know!); but the concept and consequences of, "The oxyhaemoglobin dissociation curve is shifted to the left by hypercarbia" can be expressed in a number of different ways — and, even then, the wording of the stem may alter the answer. When we think that a question is of this type we make a comment about it which you can read along with the answer: we try to point out how a question is confusing.

It is impossible to write an MCQ paper without some of the questions being ambiguous — or seeming ambiguous to some people. Some of the other questions may be ambiguous without our having realised it. We apologise for this, but some of the questions in the actual exam paper will be ambiguous, or will seem so to you in the examination hall, and you must learn how to deal with them.

It is often more difficult to think of false branches than true branches when compiling MCQ questions. Questions tend to fall into two basic types: the straightforward factual type, and the deductive type. Many pharmacology questions present facts: a drug and five properties that may or may not be properties of that drug. A false branch must appear to some candidates to be true or else the question will not discriminate between the good and poor candidate. The false branches are likely to be: the exact opposite of the true answer (eg hyperkalaemia for hypokalaemia), an association with another similar or similar-sounding drug (eg a property of chlorpropamide appended to a question on chlorpromazine), or a complete red herring. These last can be very difficult to answer, and you may not be able to find the correct answer in the literature because the connection does not exist. False answers in the deductive type of question include these types, although they may not be so obvious, but also include answers of false logic.

A Strategy for a Multiple Choice Paper

You should have a general strategy for answering an MCQ paper. For those who haven't, we suggest one here. We are not saying it is the only one, but we think it allows efficient use of the time spent answering the paper.

First, read through the questions from the first to the last answering quickly those of which you are certain of the answers. Mark the options T or F on the question paper; it is not a good idea to mark the computer card as you go because it is then not as easy to check your answers.

You will probably find that you can tell from the stem whether or not you will be able to answer a question. If you cannot answer a question immediately on this first read-through, put a question mark by it if you will need to think about it (and by any answers that you do make of which you are a little uncertain), and put a cross against those that you think you will probably not be able to answer at all. It is very important not to dwell on doubtful questions at all first time through or you may find yourself short of time before you have answered all the questions that you DO know.

On the second read-through, tackle those that you marked with a question mark; don't be afraid to scribble formulae or graphs on scrap paper to help you with confusing questions. After this second read-through it is worth going back and rechecking the answers — but don't dwell on those that you answered on the first read-through or you will find yourself doubting even your most cast-iron certainties. At this stage, transfer the answers that you have made so far to the computer cards AND MAKE SURE THAT YOU MARK THE CARDS CORRECTLY; it is easy to get out of phase between the question numbers and answer numbers. You should regard these answers as immutable: don't look at the questions again and get on with answering those that you marked with a cross. Answers to these questions you can transfer to the computer cards right away because you will have had plenty of time to think around the subject.

When you have answered all you can, check that you have written your name on everywhere that you should have done, and it may be better to leave the examination hall. With essay questions, you should always be able to add more to your answers, and you should stay for every precious minute; staying and staring at MCQ answers induces neurosis.

The MCQ Papers in this Book

The 600 questions are arranged in 10 "papers" of 60 questions. A "paper" comprises 20 questions on each of physiology, pharmacology, and physics with clinical measurement. There are 5 questions on each page: the first 4 pages of questions in each "paper" are on physiology, the middle 4 on pharmacology and the last 4 on measurement. The present format of the MCQ paper in the exam is 90 questions in 3 hours and we suggest that the best way to test yourself is to try a whole "paper" under examination conditions, unseen, in one and three-quarter hours. If you take longer than this you may run out of time in the exam when transferring your answers to the computer cards. The index at the back of the book allows access to the questions under broad subject headings so that you could, if you wanted, answer a number of questions from different papers on, say, endocrine physiology. You will, however, gain nothing if you look at the answers without trying the questions; and there is little to gain from trying a question if you have not done the work on the subject. There are more questions on some topics than on others. Some of the questions in the later papers on these important topics are similar to the questions in earlier papers and will allow you to assess whether your understanding of the topic has improved.

How to Score Yourself

For each branch, score +1 if you marked correctly True or False, or −1 if you marked incorrectly True or False. Score nil for any branch for which you gave no answer. The maximum for each question is thus +5, and the minimum is −5.

Your overall score on a "paper" will give some idea of your general level of knowledge. We cannot say what score corresponds to a "pass" in the MCQ in the actual exam, but, from our experience of setting mock papers to candidates in the past, you should be looking for 40% at the very least (60/150 for one "paper") and 60% (90/150) is a good score.

As well as your overall score it is worth calculating your "efficiency ratio", which is your number of correct answers expressed as a percentage of your total number of attempted answers. Thus you can get an overall score of 50% by answering 75 branches correctly (an efficiency of 100%) or by answering 95 but getting 10 of them wrong: $85 \times (+1)$ minus $10 \times (-1)$. A low total score with a high efficiency implies that you are certain of what you know but that your overall knowledge is not enough; a low efficiency ratio means that your knowledge is faulty, or that you are guessing.

Often, candidates going up for the exam ask how many branches they should aim to answer. The only sensible answer to this is that you should answer all that you can. There is no "safe" number. Certainly, if you are able only to answer 40%, then that is unlikely to be enough to pass, but merely ploughing on and guessing to bring your total answered up above 50% is unlikely to increase your score because half of your additional answers, if they are pure guesses, will be incorrect. Similarly, if you have answered 60%, don't assume that there is no need to answer any more — you may have answered incorrectly more than you think.

Your overall score will indicate your knowledge; your efficiency ratio will point out gross faults in technique of answering; you should also look very carefully at those individual questions at which you scored badly. Using the same reasoning as for the complete paper, you will need to score 3 out of 5 to "pass" a single question. Think carefully why you did poorly on a particular question. The usual reason is simply lack of knowledge and occasionally you will find a complete gap such that you are unable to answer any of the branches of a question. A very high negative score (-4 or -5) usually implies a lack of understanding of the question rather than lack of knowledge, or a misunderstanding of the wording. These high negative scores have a great effect on your overall score and perhaps one of the major lessons of this book is to help you to avoid them. As we have stressed before, it is essential to read each question very carefully: don't rush at the questions.

The Answers and Comments

In the answer section for each paper we give explanations of the correct answers and also make comments, if appropriate, on the form and wording of the question. It is very easy to become side-tracked and obsessed when one gets a particular branch wrong which you feel you marked correctly: you may find a source which shows you are indeed correct. However, nobody fails the MCQ paper because of one branch that, according to the "correct" answer, they answered incorrectly — concentrate instead on those questions on which you did badly overall. If you scored -3 on a question about acid-base balance it would be more valuable to go and read a good account of acid-base balance, and to seek help from others, than to feel aggrieved that you think we are wrong on one particular point and waste time laboriously checking each particular branch.

We cannot give full explanations for all the branches in all the questions: that would mean writing a large textbook. Some questions demand more explanation than others and some questions have very short comments. For many of the more important topics we advise you to consult the textbooks if you do badly. There are no references quoted, but it should be possible to answer all the questions in the book from reading of the standard texts.

The Last Word

The examiners try to set questions on sensible, mainstream, subjects that are clear and unambiguous. They are not trying to be devious and trick you into giving incorrect answers. It is often said that MCQs are unfair because they penalise the candidate who has read very widely and who can always find a reason why "true" is actually "sometimes true" or "maybe true". MCQs have to have black-or-white answers. When testing basic knowledge or general principles what the examiner wants to know is whether the candidate can see the wood for the trees.

Contents

Paper I Questions

I.1 **The following are intracellular buffers:**
  A bicarbonate and carbonic acid
  B hydroxyapatite
  C albumin
  D inorganic phosphate
  E haemoglobin.

I.2 **Autonomic ganglia:**
  A adrenaline and acetylcholine are transmitters
  B are weak autonomic centres, independent of the CNS
  C are linked to the spinal cord by grey rami communicantes
  D relay pre- to post-ganglionic impulses
  E removal of both sympathetic chains is fatal.

I.3 **These are essential amino acids:**
  A methionine
  B glycine
  C leucine
  D tyrosine
  E alanine.

I.4 **Cardiac output is increased during:**
  A stimulation of sympathetic cardiac nerves
  B tension pneumothorax
  C acclimatization to high altitude
  D hypovolaemic shock
  E stimulation of the sinus nerve.

I.5 **Pulmonary vascular resistance:**
  A is increased in hypoxia
  B is decreased by a low pH
  C can be measured using a flow-directed balloon catheter
  D is increased by isoprenaline
  E is decreased by 5-HT.

I.6   When the nerve cell membrane is suddenly depolarised, sodium permeability:

A   falls immediately to zero
B   falls only slowly, remaining low until the membrane potential is restored
C   rises immediately and is maintained at this level
D   rises only momentarily
E   is directly responsible for impulse transmission.

I.7   Sensory receptors:

A   receptor adaptation implies a decline in frequency of receptor discharge after onset of a steady stimulus
B   information is 'time-signalled' by receptors (ie interval between impulses, duration of discharge)
C   receptor information is based upon the degree of individual unit involvement
D   proprioceptors each only respond to a specific stimulus
E   stretch receptors are rapidly adapting.

I.8   One or more prostaglandins:

A   are peptides found in prostatic secretions
B   dilate the bronchi
C   stimulate uterine contractions
D   raise the intracranial pressure
E   affect platelet function.

I.9   The pituitary gland responds to secretions from the:

A   hypothalamus
B   adrenal medulla
C   adrenal cortex
D   pancreas
E   thyroid.

I.10   In the control of body temperature:

A   shivering is a spinal reflex
B   energy from brown fat is released via beta adrenergic receptors
C   brain amines play an important role
D   PGE1 may cause pyrexia
E   control is independent of higher centres.

I.11 Peristalsis in the small intestine:

A depends on an intact parasympathetic nervous system

B is coordinated by a slow wave of depolarisation

C stretch will initiate the myenteric reflex

D vasoactive intestinal peptide (VIP) is a potent inhibitor

E is inhibited by sympathetic discharge in the splanchnic nerves.

I.12 Fibrin degradation products are themselves anticoagulants interfering with:

A polymerisation of the fibrin monomer

B platelet aggregation

C thrombin activity

D serum calcium concentrations

E intrinsic pathway activation.

I.13 Pancreatic exocrine secretion:

A secretin stimulates a secretion that contains bicarbonate at concentrations that increase as the flow increases

B cholecystokinin stimulates an enzyme-rich secretion

C is not influenced by the vagus

D atropine blocks the effects of secretin and cholecystokinin

E contains a trypsin inhibitor.

I.14 Following the rapid oral ingestion of one litre of N/10 ammonium chloride solution:

A the urine will become acid

B urine output will fall

C the plasma bicarbonate will fall

D the subject will become extremely thirsty

E the ammonium ions will be converted to urea by the kidney.

I.15 Concerning renal blood flow:

A the efferent glomerular arterioles are chiefly responsible for reduction of systemic arterial pressure

B renal vasoconstriction is stimulated by a decreased baroreceptor discharge

C a 50% reduction in arterial PO_2 produces a significant reduction in renal blood flow

D renal vasodilation is a dopaminergic response

E glomerular perfusion pressure is controlled by local autoregulatory mechanisms.

I.16   In the control of respiration:

A   hypoxic drive originates in the peripheral chemoreceptors

B   there is no significant hypoxic drive in a normal subject breathing air at sea level

C   the response to CO_2 is linear over the normal range

D   the increased drive in exercise is due to incomplete oxygen equilibration in the pulmonary capillaries

E   the gasping respiration of shock is a baroreceptor reflex.

I.17   Gas content of blood:

A   the normal venous PO_2 is approximately 5.2 kPa (40 mm Hg)

B   the normal venous oxygen saturation is 75%

C   at sea level and breathing air, 0.6 ml oxygen are dissolved in 100 ml blood containing 15 gm haemoglobin/dl

D   nitrogen is only carried in arterial blood in the dissolved form

E   at a PCO_2 of 5.2 kPa (40 mm Hg) and at sea level, 47 ml CO_2 are combined with haemoglobin at a concentration of 15 gm/dl.

I.18   The following can be found in normal arterial blood:

A   5–10% carboxyhaemoglobin

B   4% methaemoglobin

C   2% free haemoglobin

D   2% foetal haemoglobin

E   25% reduced haemoglobin.

I.19   Hypoxic hypoxia:

A   can be caused by defective pulmonary oxygen transfer

B   can be caused by reduction in inspired PO_2

C   can be caused by depression of the respiratory centre

D   is unaffected by alveolar carbon dioxide concentration

E   is exacerbated by hypothermia.

I.20   The effect of hypercarbia upon the oxyhaemoglobin dissociation curve is:

A   to shift the curve to the left

B   to reduce the affinity of haemoglobin for oxygen

C   also temperature dependent

D   masked by decreases in 2,3-DPG

E   enhanced in anaemia.

I.21 The following antibiotics have a clearance greater than inulin:

A benzyl penicillin

B tetracycline

C chloramphenicol

D neomycin

E cephalexin.

I.22 Dopamine:

A increases cardiac output

B in high doses causes peripheral vasodilatation

C increases renal blood flow

D causes increased ventricular excitability

E increases splanchnic blood flow.

I.23 Atropine:

A has no effect on acetylcholine production or destruction

B 3 mg is required to produce complete vagal blockade

C is a parasympathetic depressant

D stimulates the respiratory centre

E may increase intraocular pressure.

I.24 Alpha-adrenoceptor blocking agents:

A increase blood flow in normal skin and muscle

B causes drowsiness

C all clinically useful drugs are competitive antagonists

D have only alpha1-blocking activity

E are chronotropic agents.

I.25 Procainamide:

A produces peripheral vasodilation

B has a quinidine-like myocardial effect

C is hydrolysed by pseudocholinesterase

D can only be given parenterally

E commonly produces signs of cerebral stimulation.

I.26   Diazepam:

    A   is an anticonvulsant
    B   acts on the limbic system
    C   can be metabolised to oxazepam
    D   has a half-life of less than six hours
    E   can relax skeletal muscle.

I.27   The following are aldosterone antagonists:

    A   triamterene
    B   spironolactone
    C   digitalis
    D   dopamine
    E   diazoxide.

I.28   The following are bronchodilators:

    A   salbutamol
    B   sodium chromoglycate
    C   noradrenaline
    D   doxapram
    E   theophylline.

I.29   Metyrapone:

    A   is used therapeutically in mild cases of Cushing's syndrome
    B   inhibits the production of both cortisol and aldosterone
    C   results in increased corticotrophin levels
    D   must be given intravenously
    E   a response is measured by urinary 17-oxogenic steroids.

I.30   The following statements are true:

    A   methoxyflurane is very soluble in rubber
    B   the blood/gas partition coeffient of isoflurane is 1.4
    C   chloroform is a relatively soluble agent
    D   enflurane is a halogenated hydrocarbon
    E   the vapour pressure of ether at 20°C is 57 kPa.

I.31 **Etomidate:**
  A induces epilepsy
  B is metabolised by Hoffman elimination
  C produces immunologically-mediated hypersensitivity reactions
  D possesses analgesic properties
  E is soluble in water.

I.32 **A base with a pK of 9:**
  A will be strongly ionised in the stomach
  B will be 75% ionised at a pH of 4.5
  C would be better excreted in an acid urine
  D will prevent the uptake of salicylate
  E will be strongly protein bound.

I.33 **Thiopentone:**
  A at normal plasma pH, is 50–75% bound to plasma proteins
  B is a thiosubstituted succinylurea
  C in 2.5% solution it has a pH greater than 10
  D after re-distribution, it is rapidly metabolised in the liver
  E its excretion is usefully accelerated by a forced alkaline diuresis.

I.34 **Perphenazine:**
  A is a phenothiazine
  B precipitates oculogyric crises
  C should not be given in pregnancy
  D produces mild alpha adrenergic blockade
  E acts on the chemoreceptor trigger zone.

I.35 **Insulin:**
  A increases formation of both liver and muscle glycogen
  B inhibits gluconeogenesis
  C reduces protein synthesis
  D lowers serum potassium concentration
  E increases fat synthesis.

I.36   **Methods of prolonging the duration of action of lignocaine include:**

   A   the addition of adrenaline
   B   carbonation
   C   using a more concentrated solution
   D   mixing with dextran in saline
   E   increasing the volume of drug injected.

I.37   **Pseudocholinesterase:**

   A   is found in plasma
   B   is inhibited by organophosphorus compounds
   C   plasma levels are reduced during pregnancy
   D   is stimulated by fluoride ions
   E   is responsible for the inactivation of succinylcholine.

I.38   **Cocaine:**

   A   competes with noradrenaline at binding sites
   B   may produce vomiting
   C   depresses respiration
   D   hypersensitivity is rare
   E   is largely excreted unchanged in urine.

I.39   **Pentazocine:**

   A   produces a similar degree of respiratory depression to that induced by an equipotent dose of pethidine
   B   is chemically incompatible with diazepam
   C   induces respiratory depression reversed by naloxone
   D   can be used to reverse fentanyl induced respiratory depression
   E   may induce confusion in the elderly.

I.40   **The following interfere with blood grouping or incompatability testing:**

   A   dextran 40
   B   warfarin
   C   dipyridamole
   D   aspirin
   E   tranexamic acid.

I.41 **A plot of pressure against volume:**

    A allows compliance to be measured

    B may show hysteresis

    C allows a direct measurement of airways resistance

    D is usually plotted on semi-logarithmic paper

    E allows an estimate to be made of respiratory work.

I.42 **In the cryoprobe:**

    A cooling is an adiabatic process

    B rapid gas expansion from a capillary tube produces a fall in temperature

    C cooling is due to energy loss resulting from gas expansion

    D carbon dioxide is a suitable gas for routine use

    E tip temperatures as low as $-90°C$ are required for efficient use.

I.43 **Concerning gas chromatography:**

    A the stationary phase is usually silica-alumina coated with polyethylene glycol

    B the carrier gas is usually nitrogen or helium

    C solubility of the individual substances in the stationary phase is temperature dependent

    D in a flame ionisation detector, a polarising voltage is applied across the flame of ionised particles and the magnitude of the current produced is dependent upon the nature of the particles in the flame

    E none of the detectors used allow absolute identification of the separated compounds without prior calibration.

I.44 **Clinical trials:**

    A are said to be single-blind when only the subject is unaware of the treatment used

    B are said to be double-blind when neither the physicians or subjects are aware of which treatment is being used

    C single-blind trials do not require the use of a placebo

    D sequential analysis is unsuitable for a double-blind study

    E observer bias may still occur in a double-blind trial.

I.45 **In the ECG at a heart rate of 80 per minute:**

    A the PR interval should be less than 0.2 and greater than 0.12 sec

    B the QRS complex should last less than 0.02 sec

    C the T wave is normally greater than 1 mV

    D there should be an interval of 0.75 seconds between the end of one complex and the beginning of the next

    E the T wave is ventricular repolarisation.

I.46   Which of the following statements are true:

- **A** the null hypothesis states that there is nothing to be gained from treatment
- **B** the significance level is a probability value that ensures that the outcome is clinically significant
- **C** the standard deviation is a measure of the central value of the sample
- **D** the standard error is the measure of the precision of an estimate in relation to its unknown true value in the population
- **E** blood pressure is measured on an ordinal scale.

I.47   Rise in alveolar concentration of anaesthetic agents is faster:

- **A** when the inspired concentration is higher
- **B** when the alveolar ventilation is increased
- **C** when the cardiac output is increased
- **D** when the agent is more soluble
- **E** when nitrous oxide is added to the inspired mixture.

I.48   Compared with intracellular fluid, the extracellular fluid contains a greater concentration of:

- **A** sodium ions
- **B** magnesium ions
- **C** protein
- **D** hydrogen ions
- **E** bicarbonate ions.

I.49   The following are true:

- **A** the plasma osmotic pressure is 7 atmospheres
- **B** osmolality is osmols per kilogram of solvent
- **C** osmolality can be measured by depression of melting point of a liquid
- **D** the mathematical description of osmosis is analogous to the gas laws
- **E** osmosis is generated by contact between differing concentrations of a solute.

I.50   An electromanometer can be based on:

- **A** the fuel cell
- **B** variable capacitance
- **C** variable inductance
- **D** the Wheatstone bridge
- **E** variable conductance.

I.51 **pH can be measured with:**
  A   a siver-silver chloride bridge electrode
  B   a mercury half cell
  C   a calomel half cell
  D   a glass electrode
  E   a platinum electrode.

I.52 **Concerning location of vaporisers within the anaesthetic circuit:**
  A   with the vaporiser inside a circle (VIC), the inflow gas contains an unknown concentration of volatile agent
  B   with VIC an accurate vaporiser, efficierit at low flows should be used to maintain an accurate vapour concentration within the circuit
  C   with the vaporiser outside the circle (VOC) an ineffient vaporiser is indicated because inspired concentrations are not critical
  D   with VOC the anaesthetic vapour concentration within the circuit is dependent upon uptake
  E   with VIC and low fresh gas flow, the inspired concentration is greater than the vaporiser setting.

I.53 **The following are true:**
  A   a catheter of 28 FG will have a circumference of 28 mm
  B   a needle of 21 SWG is larger than one of 23 SWG
  C   a cannula of 14 SWG external diameter will allow a maximum flow of one litre in about 4 minutes
  D   an endotracheal tube size 8 will have an external diameter of 8 mm
  E   the standard BS tapers are 15, 22 and 32 mm.

I.54 **Methods used to measure CO_2 in a mixture of gases include:**
  A   katharometer
  B   manometric van Slyke apparatus
  C   Haldane apparatus
  D   infra red gas analyzer
  E   Severinghaus electrode.

I.55 **The following are flammable:**
  A   ethyl chloride
  B   0.5% chlorhexidine in 70% alcohol
  C   trichloroethylene
  D   nitrous oxide at high temperatures
  E   fluoroxene.

I.56   Critical temperature:

    A critical temperature is the temperature above which a substance cannot be liquified however much pressure is applied

    B the critical temperature of oxygen is −119°C

    C nitrous oxide cylinders always contain liquid nitrous oxide

    D the critical temperature of nitrous oxide is 48.5°C *(36·5)*

    E critical pressure is the vapour pressure of a substance at its critical temperature.

I.57   In the Astrup interpolation method of blood gas analysis:

    A the buffer line for a particular blood sample in obtained by tonometry with two different carbon dioxide concentrations

    B the only direct measurement made is that of pH

    C the mercury reference electrode is linked to a potassium chloride solution through a porous plug

    D derived values, including buffer base are obtained by plotting pH against PCO_2 on a Siggaard-Anderson nomogram

    E phosphate buffers of standard pH are used for spanning the pH electrode.

I.58   Solubility:

    A the Ostwald solubility coefficient is independent of pressure

    B for the Ostwald solubility coefficient, the volume of gas is measured at ambient temperature and pressure

    C the partition coefficient is defined as the ratio of the amount of substance present in one phase compared with another.

    D the tension of a gas in solution is the partial pressure of the gas which would be in equilibrium with it

    E partition coefficients are temperature specific.

I.59   Surface tension:

    A is measured as Newtons per square metre

    B at the junction of fluid and the wall of a tube, surface tension acts vertically as well as horizontally

    C the pressure generated by surface tension in a sphere is double that in a tubular structure

    D Laplace's law for a sphere states that the transmural pressure is directly proportional to twice the surface tension and to the radius of the sphere

    E surface tension is a direct result of molecular attraction at the surface of the liquid.

I.60   For an exponential process with a negative exponent:

    A the time constant is the natural logarithm of the half-life

    B the rate of the process is highest at the beginning

    C a plot on semi-logarithmic paper will give a straight line

    D an example would be unaided, passive exhalation

    E it always takes the same time to reach half its current value.

Paper I Answers

I.1   TTFFT

A   The bicarbonate system is much more important as an extracellular buffer, but the answer must be "true" because of the red blood cell.

B   In bone.

C   Albumin is an extracellular buffer.

D   Organic phosphates are intracellular buffers.

E   Via the imidazole groups of the histidine residues.

I.2   FFFTF

A   Acetylcholine only.

C   True for sympathetic ganglia, but not all.

E   Not directly.

I.3   TFTFF

D   Tyrosine is non-essential unless phenylalanine is missing from the diet.

I.4   TFTFF

B   Compression of the heart and great veins reduces venous return.

D   In shock caused solely by hypovolaemia, the shock results from the failure of cardiac output.

E   Baroreceptor afferents = high blood pressure, cardiac output will fall to correct it.

I.5   TFTFF

C   To know the resistance one must know the pressure differential and the flow: both can be measured with the catheter.

E   The effect of 5-HT on smooth muscle is complex: there will be vasocon– striction or vasodilation depending on the particular vascular bed, the resting tone, and the dose. There are also effects via reflexes, by affecting ganglionic transmission, etc. The pulmonary vascular resistance increases sharply in dogs and cats, but less so in man.

I.6   FFFFT

A,B,C,D   Bad question – mutually exclusive options. Sodium permeability rises slightly during the local depolarisation response and then when the firing level is reached, sodium permeability rises sharply.

I.7   TTTTF

E   Slowly adapting.

I.8   FTTFT

The prostaglandins are unsaturated fatty acids (not peptides). They have a great variety of actions in many tissues and it would be foolish to try and learn them all. They are now used clinically (e.g. **C**, **E**, and also to prevent closure of the ductus) and clinically useful actions you should certainly know.

A   They are found in seminal vesicle fluid.

I.9   TFTFT

B   Negative feedback from cortex.
D   Pancreatic secretions are controlled by locally released hormones, eg secretin, pancreozymin.

I.10   FTTTF

A   Shivering depends on central coordination.
B   In humans, brown fat is found only in infants.
C   There are species differences; 5-hydroxytryptamine and nor-adrenaline have been implicated.
E   Temperature causes changes in behaviour, e.g. moving into the shade on a very hot day.

I.11   **FTTFT**

A   An intact myenteric nerve plexus is required.

B   A wave moves through the longitudinal muscle about 10 times per minute.

C   The myenteric reflex initiates a peristaltic wave.

D   VIP is a regulator of secretion. The use of the adjective "potent" means that **D** will remain false even if someone somewhere describes an effect of VIP on an isolated segment of bowel in an experiment. Remember that this exam is concerned with a good understanding of the basic principles, not with the minutiae of "state of the art" research.

E   This causes the reflex ileus of peritoneal irritation.

I.12   **TTTFF**

D,E   No evidence that FDP's interfere with either of these mechanisms.

I.13   **TTFFT**

C,D   Vagal stimulation increases enzyme-rich secretion: this effect, but not the effects of the hormones, are blocked by atropine.

E   Like other systems in which precursors are converted to active forms, eg the coagulation cascade, inhibitors are present to maintain a balance and prevent runaway positive feedback.

I.14   **TFTFF**

A   Ammonium chloride is an acidifying salt that can be used, in suitable combination with other electrolyte solutions, in severe metabolic alkalosis.

B   It is a diuretic, increasing urine output by supplying an acid load.

D   The diuresis is not that severe, and ammonium chloride has no specific property of inducing thirst.

E   Conversion of ammonium to urea occurs in the liver.

I.15   **TTTTF**

E   No local mechanisms involved – alterations in renal perfusion occur in response to central effects related to hypertension, hypoxia, etc.

I.16   TFTFF
- **B**   Breathing 100% oxygen at sea-level depresses respiration.
- **D**   There are many inputs in exercise. Oxygen equilibration will be complete unless exercise is severe, or there is anaemia, or there is a block to diffusion.
- **E**   Hypoxia and acidosis at the chemoreceptors.

I.17   TTFTF
- **C**   0.3 ml – 3 ml/litre.
- **E**   The figure is correct but for the TOTAL CO_2 in the blood not the amount combined with haemoglobin.

I.18   FFFTF
- **A**   These concentrations may be found in the blood of heavy smokers.
- **B**   It does form in normal man but is reduced by NADH-metHb reductase system.
- **C**   Haemoglobin is not found free in the circulation: it is nephrotoxic.
- **E**   25% reduced Hb is equivalent to a PaO_2 of 40 mm Hg, ie venous blood.

I.19   TTTTF
- **E**   Hypothermia shifts oxyhaemoglobin dissociation curve to the left, reducing oxygen delivery and maintaining arterial oxygen content. Hypothermia also reduces oxygen utilisation and demand.

I.20   FTTTT
- **A**   Hypercarbia and acidosis shift curve to right.
- **C**   True, curve is temperature dependent whatever position it is in.
- **D**   True, decreases in 2,3-DPG shift curve to left, hypercarbia shifts it in the opposite direction

I.21 **TFTFT**

A clearance greater than that of inulin implies active tubular secretion; this is so for penicillin (**A**) and cephalexin (**E**).

C Unaltered chloramphenicol is excreted by glomerular filtration, but the inactive degradation products are secreted by the tubules.

I.22 **TFTTT**

A It is both inotropic and chronotropic.
B In high doses it is an alpha-agonist.
C,E There are specific dopaminergic receptors that subserve vasodilation in the kidney and mesentery.

I.23 **TTTTT**

D Is a general cerebral stimulant.
E By producing mydriasis but, at least with normal clinical doses, only when applied topically.

I.24 **TTFFF**

A It will depend on the prevailing sympathetic tone.
C Phenoxybenzamine is not a competitive inhibitor.
D Sub-division of alpha-receptors is not as clear, not are the clinical implications so obvious, as the sub-division of beta-receptors. Alpha– blocking agents, as a group, are not selective.
E Although they may cause a reflex tachycardia.

I.25 **TTFFF**

C Unlike procaine, this does not occur to a significant extent.
D Can also be given orally.
E Much less than with procaine.

I.26   TTTFT

    B   The benzodiazepines affect the hippocampus, and other areas, quite selectively.

    C   Diazepam CAN be metabolised to oxazepam but it is via an intermediate, is species-specific, and oxazepam has a shorter half-life than diazepam. It is of more importance to know when a drug is metabolised to a product that has a longer half-life (eg thiopentone to pentobarbitone).

    D   20–90 hrs (oxazepam, incidentally, is 3–21 hrs).

    E   Not by a direct action but by actions at supraspinal loci.

I.27   TTFFF

    C   Diuretic effect related to increased renal perfusion.

    D   Separate effect on dopaminergic receptors.

    E   Not a diuretic.

I.28   TFFFT

    A   Beta–2 stimulation.

    B   It does not directly cause dilatation, it stabilises mast cell membranes and so reduces histamine release.

    C   Nor-adrenaline is an alpha-agonist.

    D   Doxapram is effectively a centrally acting respiratory stimulant, though there is evidence it acts on the peripheral arterial chemoreceptors.

I.29   FTTFT

Metyrapone is a competitive inhibitor of 11 beta-hydroxylation in the synthesis of steroids and is used in the diagnosis of adrenocorticoid disorders.

    A   No, although it can be used in Cushing's syndrome when associated with carcinoma that is not amenable to surgery.

    C   Because the feedback loop is broken.

    D   It can be given orally.

I.30   TTTFT

    A   Agents usually have similar solubilities in rubber and fat. During induction with methoxyflurane, very little agent actually reaches the patient to begin with.

    D   A halogenated ether.

I.31   FFFFF
 A Not epileptogenic.
 B Hoffman elimination is related to atracurium.
 C The only documented reactions are related to direct
   histamine release but these are rare.
 E Propylene glycol.

I.32   TFTFF
 An important topic that results in questions that can be
 confusing because of the wording. Try to think it through
 logically: pK is the pH at 50% ionisation, and acids tend to ionise
 in solutions of relative alkalinity (and vice versa).
 D,E One cannot predict these merely from knowing the pK.

I.33   TFTFF
 B Malonyl urea.
 D Metabolised, but only at 10–15% per hour.
 E Theoretically "true" because it is a weak acid, but usefully
   or clinically "false".

I.34   TTFTT
 C Phenothiazine anti-emetics are not contraindicated in
   pregnancy.

I.35   TTFTT
 B True, insulin inhibits gluconeogenesis and ketogenesis.
 C Increases protein synthesis.

I.36   TTTTT
>   **B**   Exposing the solution to carbon dioxide alters the pH and therefore the rate of membrane transfer of the drug.
>   **C,E**   Both are true for epidural application though probably not for local nerve blocks.

I.37   TTTFT
>   **B**   Includes insecticides and "nerve gases". Their main action is on acetylcholinesterase but they also inactivate other esterases.
>   **D** F^- is a differential inhibitor, used in the diagnosis of atypical enzyme.

I.38   TTFFF
>   **C**   Respiratory rate increased, but depth unaffected.
>   **D**   Common – many people routinely test for hypersensitivity.
>   **E**   Mainly metabolised, but a small amount is excreted unchanged.

I.39   TTFTT
>   **C**   May induce respiratory depression, but this is only reversible in a non-specific way by analeptic drugs such as doxapram.

I.40   TFFFF
>   **A**   All dextrans interfere, particularly those of high molecular weight.
>   **B,C,D,E**   All affect coagulation, but not cross-matching.
>   **E**   Mefenamic acid interferes.

Methyl dopa and high dose penicillin are two other common drugs that may interfere.

I.41   TTFFT

B   ie the relation between pressure and volume is different if the pressure is increasing from when it is decreasing: the plot will then show a "hysteresis loop."

C   Resistance implies flow, which includes the time: there is no direct measure of time on a pressure-volume loop.

E   Work = force × distance. Application of algebra to this equation and your knowledge of the meaning of pressure and volume should show that work = pressure × volume.

I.42   TTTTF

B   The principle of the cryoprobe is that gas expands rapidly after leaving a capillary tube and produces a fall in temperature.

D   Although nitrous oxide is often used, carbon dioxide is equally suitable.

E   Maximum tip temperature achievable is –70°C.

I.43   TTTTT

C   True, the column is heated to drive off adsorbed substances.

I.44   TTFFT

C   Degree of blindness does not effect the need for a placebo.

D   Sequential analysis is simply used as a comparison between two alternatives and is still suitable for a double-blind study

E   True – particularly if a particular parameter, e.g. respiration rate is being observed.

I.45   TFFFT

B   Up to 0.1 sec.

D   Work it out: rate 80 × interval 0.75 sec = 60 secs. There wouldn't be any time for the complexes between the intervals

I.46   FFFTT

A   The null hypothesis is that the samples being tested are from the same population: it is a statistical, not a clinical, statement.

B   Only states that the outcome is statistically significant.

C   Is a measure of the variability.

I.47   TTFFT

C   Rise in alveolar concentration is faster when cardiac output is reduced, increased output removes gas quicker.

D   A soluble drug passes into blood more readily and therefore the alveolar partial pressure takes longer to rise.

I.48   TFFFT

	ICF	ECF
Na	12	145
Mg	15	2
Prot	60	16
pH	7.0	7.4
HCO_3	8	27

I.49   TTTTF

A   This is the total osmotic pressure; oncotic pressure is the effective osmotic pressure and is much less (30 mm Hg).

B   Osmolarity is per litre of solution.

D   ie PV=nRT.

E   Only if the membrane separating the concentrations is impermeable to the solute.

I.50   FTTTT

An electromanometer can be made using any electrical var

A   The fuel cell is the basis for a method of measuring oxygen.

A   A Wheatstone bridge is a circuit of resistances that can be balanced for nil current flow.

I.51   FFFTF

The mercury and calomel half-cells are constituents of electrode systems; silver-silver chloride and platinum electrodes are used for recording various biological potentials. Only the glass electrode can measure pH. You must know the theory and structure of pH electrodes.

I.52   FFFTT

A   With VIC the inflow gas (FGF) contains no volatile agent.
B,C   These are each stated opposite to the true answer.

I.53   TTTFF

A,B,C FG = French gauge. SWG = steel wire gauge.
C   The flow will depend on the internal, not the external, diameter. Nonetheless, this is a realistic figure for such a cannula (actually the quoted rate from a 14G Venflon).
D   Internal diameter.
E   These are the tapers on anaesthetic circuits: 15 and 22 are correct, but the exhaust taper is 30 mm.

I.54   TFTTT

A   The katharometer can have a response fast enough for breath-by-breath analysis.
B   For gas in blood: but it is difficult, time-consuming, and inaccurate in the presence of anaesthetic gases.
C   A modification of the Haldane apparatus is still the absolute standard by which more sophisticated equipment is calibrated.

I.55   TTTFT

B   An important source of fire and morbidity is pools of spirit solutions under the operative drapes.
C   It will not burn under normal conditions.
D   Nitrous oxide is neither flammable nor explosive but it supports combustion at temperatures above 450°C when it starts to break down to nitrogen and oxygen.

1.56   TTFFT

C   They only contain liquid nitrous oxide before all the liquid becomes vaporised and when not in very hot conditions.
D   36.5°C.

1.57   TTTTT

A   Although not used now, this forms the basis for current methods of performing and interpreting blood gas analysis and is often asked.

1.58   TTFTT

C   The definition includes the two phases being of equal volume and being in equilibrium.

1.59   FTTFT

A   It is force per unit length, ie Newtons per metre.
D   P= 2T/R; inversely proportional to radius. Note that **C** and **D** can't both be true.

1.60   FTTTT

Time constant and half-life are two ways of describing the rate of an exponential process. The half-life is easier to understand and is stated in **E**. The time constant is about one and a half times the half-life and is best understood from a consideration of the mathematics of the exponential process; it is also the time in which the process would be completed if it were to continue at its initial rate.

Paper II Questions

II.1 **Compensatory mechanisms for a primary acidosis include:**
- **A** hyperventilation
- **B** increased urine pH
- **C** elevated CSF bicarbonate
- **D** decreased carbonic anhydrase activity within the renal tubular cells
- **E** bicarbonate excretion to control urine pH.

II.2 **Sympathetic innervation of blood vessels:**
- **A** is an alpha adrenergic effect
- **B** is mediated locally by noradrenaline
- **C** sympathectomy induces vasodilation
- **D** sympathectomy produces no effect on vessel diameter, but flow is increased
- **E** induces vasodilation in response to cold and haemorrhage.

II.3 **In protein metabolism:**
- **A** methionine is a common source of methyl groups for synthesis
- **B** the urea cycle involves ornithine, citrulline and arginine
- **C** the urea cycle produces both urea and uric acid
- **D** creatinine is synthesised directly from creatine
- **E** essential amino acids are L-forms, non-essential are D-forms.

II.4 **Venous return is decreased by:**
- **A** ganglion-blocking drugs
- **B** exercise
- **C** paralysis of skeletal muscles
- **D** femoral arterio-venous fistula
- **E** rapid infusion of blood.

II.5 **In the normal cardiac cycle:**
- **A** the period of ventricular systole is equal to the Q-T interval
- **B** the duration of the QRS complex depends on the heart rate
- **C** the PR interval is less than 0.22 secs
- **D** ejection occurs throughout systole
- **E** the R-R interval varies.

II.6   Nerve conduction:

A   at the height of the action potential the membrane potential approaches the equilibrium potential balancing the ions on the two sides of the membrane

B   the duration of the absolute refractory period is less than 10 msec

C   the length of the refractory period limits transmission frequency

D   is fastest in myelinated fibres

E   saltatory conduction involves sodium and chloride permeability alone.

II.7   Potassium balance:

A   is acutely regulated by changes in concentration across cell membranes

B   plasma levels are acutely elevated by an alpha adrenergic affect

C   hyperkalaemia increases insulin secretion

D   hyperkalaemia decreases glucagon secretion

E   intracellular alkalosis decreases serum potassium.

II.8   Insulin has the following actions in skeletal muscle:

A   enhances glycogen synthesis

B   enhances uptake of amino acids

C   increases protein synthesis

D   increases production of ketones

E   increases phosphorylation of glucose.

II.9   Antidiuretic hormone:

A   is produced in the posterior lobe of the pituitary gland

B   release is stimulated by a rise in plasma osmolality

C   release is stimulated by an increase in effective ECF volume

D   inappropriate release may occur during surgery

E   is also a vasoconstrictor in physiological concentrations.

II.10   Serum albumin:

A   is synthesised mainly in the reticuloendothelial system

B   has a half-life in the circulation of approximately 3 days

C   is generally normal in acute liver disease

D   is 5–10% higher in the recumbent than in the upright position

E   is increased 10–20% after prolonged venous stasis.

II.11 **Deficiences of the following cause specific faults in erythropoiesis:**
   A ascorbic acid
   B folic acid
   C vitamin E
   D cyanocobalamin (B12)
   E valine.

II.12 **Haematological changes in pathological fibrinolysis include:**
   A reduced concentrations of plasminogen
   B fibrin degradation product concentration greater than 10
   C increased fibrinogen concentrations
   D haemoglobinuria
   E increased concentration of plasminogen activator.

II.13 **Cerebrospinal fluid:**
   A has a higher glucose content than blood
   B has a better buffering capacity than blood
   C the normal cell count is 50 – 100 per cubic millimetre
   D is a clear yellow liquid
   E has a lower pH than blood.

II.14 **In the nephron:**
   A all membranes are equally permeable to water, gradients develop because of membrane ionic pumps
   B two-thirds of the glomerular filtrate is absorbed in the proximal convoluted tubule
   C the medulla has an osmolarity of 1200 mOsm/L
   D sodium is exchanged for potassium in the distal convoluted tubule
   E the collecting ducts form a countercurrent multiplier.

II.15 **Renin:**
   A secretion occurs from the juxta-glomerular cells around the afferent glomerular arterioles
   B release occurs in response to a decrease in mean renal arterial blood pressure
   C release occurs in response to changes in sodium and chloride delivery to the kidney
   D release is important in the maintenance of blood pressure under ether anaesthesia
   E release is significantly increased under halothane anaesthesia.

II.16　At high altitude, pulmonary ventilation increase because:

A　the barometric pressure is lower
B　alveolar PCO_2 falls
C　it is an adapation to raise the alveolar PO_2
D　oxygen consumption increases
E　pulmonary oedema develops.

II.17　The oxygen capacity of the blood is:

A　the maximum quantity of oxygen which will combine with 100 ml whole blood at BTPS
B　the ratio between oxygen uptake and pH in the blood
C　is independent of the haemoglobin concentration
D　only refers to oxygen physically dissolved in blood
E　is normally of the order of 15–18 volumes per 100 ml whole blood.

II.18　In acute hypoxia:

A　dyspnoea combined with hyperpnoea is diagnostic
B　there is tachycardia
C　the blood pressure is high
D　respiratory stimulation is from the peripheral chemoreceptors
E　there will be cyanosis.

II.19　The following statements are true of the oxyhaemoglobin dissociation curve:

A　the p50 is approximately 3.6 kPa (27 mm Hg)
B　the curve moves to the right if there is hypercarbia
C　the curve moves to the left if there is acidaemia
D　the p50 is decreased by a raised $PaCO_2$
E　the steepest part of the curve is below the normal venous point.

II.20　At functional residual capacity:

A　a healthy subject should be able to breath-hold for at least 25 seconds
B　the tendency of the chest wall to expand is exactly balanced by the tendency of the lungs to collapse
C　ventilation-perfusion ratios are optimal
D　static compliance is minimal
E　the lungs still contain the expiratory reserve volume and the residual volume.

II.21   Aminoglycoside antibiotics:
- **A**   cannot be given orally
- **B**   are active against Staph. aureus
- **C**   are useful in severe infections presumed to be due to Ps. aeruginosa
- **D**   should be avoided in pregnancy
- **E**   excretion is 60% renal, 40% metabolised.

II.22   Heart rate is slowed by:
- **A**   amphetamine
- **B**   atropine
- **C**   propranolol
- **D**   dobutamine
- **E**   nifedipine.

II.23   Atropine:
- **A**   reduces the oxygen saturation of arterial blood
- **B**   reduces physiological dead space
- **C**   can induce hyperpyrexia in children
- **D**   increases the incidence of halothane induced dysrhythmias
- **E**   increases the likelihood of regurgitation on induction.

II.24   Using propranolol to treat hypertension:
- **A**   exacerbates asthma
- **B**   often produces postural hypotension
- **C**   is contra-indicated in patients with high plasma renin levels
- **D**   may precipitate cardiac failure in susceptible patients
- **E**   should be avoided in a patient with Raynaud's phenomenon.

II.25   Methoxamine:
- **A**   is a pure alpha stimulant
- **B**   has both direct and indirect effects at adrenergic receptors
- **C**   increases the irritability of heart muscle
- **D**   decreases cardiac output
- **E**   should only be given intravenously.

II.26   The following are anti-convulsants:

    A   methohexitone
    B   suxamethonium
    C   chlormethiazole
    D   thiopentone
    E   lignocaine.

II.27   Diazoxide:

    A   is a diuretic
    B   produces salt and water retention
    C   has a hypotensive effect
    D   does not impair glucose tolerance
    E   is not protein bound.

II.28   Sodium nitroprusside infusion:

    A   is used for the long term medical management of dissecting aneurysm of the aorta
    B   causes dilated pupils
    C   is metabolised by liver rhodanese
    D   can result in persistent lactic acidosis
    E   causes reflex stimulation of the parasympathetic nervous system.

II.29   The following drugs will stimulate vasopressin secretion:

    A   morphine
    B   carbamazepine
    C   alcohol
    D   chlorpropamide
    E   dipyridamole.

II.30   Methohexitone:

    A   is more potent than thiopentone
    B   can cause pain on injection
    C   can cause excitatory movements
    D   is an anticonvulsant
    E   is unstable in solution.

II.31 **Halothane:**
- **A** has a boiling point of 104°C
- **B** has a saturated vapour pressure at 20°C of 243 mm Hg
- **C** is relatively insoluble in blood compared with other anaesthetic vapours
- **D** can be used with aluminium apparatus
- **E** is stable on exposure to light.

II.32 **A drug that is strongly protein bound:**
- **A** will be metabolised rapidly
- **B** interferes with the pharmacodynamics of warfarin
- **C** will induce liver enzymes
- **D** will cause an increase in the serum albumin
- **E** will have a relatively low "free" level in the plasma.

II.33 **The following are isotonic:**
- **A** 20% mannitol
- **B** 5% dextrose
- **C** 0.9M NaCl
- **D** Hartmann's solution (Ringer-Lactate)
- **E** HPPF.

II.34 **Which of the following are true:**
- **A** alkalinisation of the urine increases the excretion of phenobarbitone
- **B** acidification of the urine reduces aspirin elimination
- **C** hydrogen ion excretion in the kidney is dependant upon carbonic anhydrase activity
- **D** acetazolamide therapy may produce hypokalaemia
- **E** elective hyperventilation reduces hydrogen ion excretion.

II.35 **Mono-amine oxidase:**
- **A** is ineffective in the breakdown of histamine
- **B** is inhibited by ephedrine
- **C** is produced in the placenta
- **D** the highest concentration in the body occurs in the brain
- **E** is physiologically responsible for intraneuronal metabolism of noradrenline which has leaked from storage granules.

II.36   Central effects of lignocaine include:

A   sedation
B   convulsions
C   vomiting
D   tachycardia
E   tinnitus.

II.37   Tubocurarine:

A   will block autonomic ganglia
B   is antagonised by magnesium ions
C   does not cause histamine release
D   is partially inactivated before excretion
E   crosses the placenta.

II.38   Acetylcholinesterase:

A   is present in red blood cells
B   the anionic site binds the N^+ atom of acetylcholine
C   hydrolysis of acetylcholine produces acetylation of the enzyme
D   is inhibited by acid-transfer from neostigmine
E   acetylation of the enzyme under physiological conditions may persist for several hours.

II.39   Narcotic antagonists:

A   nalorphine will not counteract fentanyl-induced respiratory depression
B   naloxone precipitates hypertension
C   naloxone can be used in the treatment of morphine addiction
D   excessive treatment with nalorphine will potentiate morphine-induced respiratory depression
E   the addition of levallorphan to pethidine increases the likelihood of undesired side effects.

II.40   The following have interactions likely to be of clinical importance:

A   propranolol and ergotamine
B   metformin and alcohol
C   pancuronium and carbenicillin
D   tolbutamide and sulphinpyrazone
E   oral iron and chloramphenicol.

II.41 Methods of measuring cardiac output include:

A thermodilution
B electromagnetic flow meter
C impedance of the chest wall
D limb plethysmography
E radio-isotopes.

II.42 Biological potentials:

A the normal signal amplitude of the ECG is of the order of 1–2 mV
B recordings are normally a display of the difference in potential of two electrodes
C the frequency distribution of the ECG signal is between 0.5 and 80 Hz
D the EMG may cause interference on the ECG because similar potentials are involved
E the EEG does not interfere with the ECG.

II.43 Gas chromatography is used in the measurement of:

A halothane
B barbiturates
C benzodiazepines
D nitrous oxide in blood
E catecholamines.

II.44 The electromagnetic spectrum:

A because the velocity of the waves in the spectrum is constant, the individual wavelengths are proportional to the reciprocal of the frequency
B the frequency of X-rays and gamma rays is between 10^{-18} and 10^{-21}
C the wavelength of ultraviolet is longer than that of infra-red light
D radio waves have a lower frequency than X-rays
E gases are capable of absorbing electromagnetic radiation.

II.45 The closing volume:

A increases with age
B always includes the FRC
C is higher when supine than when upright
D is measured by forced expiration after a full inspiration of a marker gas
E is indicated on the tracer-volume curve at the transition between phases III and IV.

II.46 Which of the following statements are true:

A   the unpaired 't' test is a test of the difference of sample means

B   the 't' test was described by a mathematics student

C   the Chi-squared test can only be used on nominal data

D   if a drug produces no statistical difference between two samples it can be concluded that it is ineffective

E   correlation measures association but not causation.

II.47 The Henderson-Hasselbalch equation:

A   implies that there is a constant ratio between CO_2 and bicarbonate

B   is usually calculated from data obtained in vivo

C   uses a pK of approximately 6.1

D   this pK changes with temperature

E   includes a term for buffer base.

II.48 In the measurement of renal function:

A   inulin is used because it is completely cleared by the glomeruli

B   creatinine clearance is approximately the same as inulin clearance

C   glomerular filtration is inversely proportional to the blood urea

D   up to 150 mg of protein may be lost daily through normal kidneys

E   the normal serum creatinine is less than 133 micromol/L.

II.49 The following are true of osmosis:

A   it is the basis of the red cell fragility test

B   the osmolarity of body fluids is approximately 290 mOsmol/L, mainly due to proteins

C   large molecules are more efficient generators of osmotic pressure

D   oncotic pressure is the effective osmotic pressure of the plasma and is approximately 4 kPa (30 mm Hg)

E   the pressure can be calculated by using Raoult's law.

II.50 When recording an electrical signal:

A   digital meters usually have a faster response than those with a moving needle

B   electrical filters always reduce the signal to noise ratio

C   the frequency response of a suitable recorder should be linear to about the 10th harmonic of the fundamental

D   matching of equipment impedances is important

E   zero stability may depend on temperature.

II.51 **When measuring arterial blood pressure using a sphygmomanometer cuff:**
- **A** if the cuff is too small for the arm the pressure will tend to read high
- **B** accuracy is increased by leaving the cuff slightly inflated between readings
- **C** the slower the deflation, the more accurate the reading
- **D** a mercury column will have a low frequency response
- **E** diastolic pressure will agree more accurately with direct measurement than will systolic pressure.

II.52 **Nerve stimulator:**
- **A** the electrical potential involved can be as high as 150 volts
- **B** the tetanic stimulus is at a set frequency of 50 Hz
- **C** the train-of-four uses a pulse duration of 200 msec and a frequency of 2 Hz
- **D** higher electrical potentials are necessary if subcutaneous electrodes are used
- **E** the apparatus uses a square wave electrical signal.

II.53 **Concerning a ventilator that is a flow generator and time-cycled:**
- **A** the respiratory frequency is independent of the tidal volume
- **B** it will, within limits, deliver a given tidal volume however the resistance of the airways changes
- **C** the tidal volume will depend on the compliance
- **D** the pressure generated in the upper airways will depend on the resistance and compliance of the chest
- **E** the I:E ratio will be fixed at a given respiratory frequency.

II.54 **One gram molecular weight of any gas:**
- **A** contains the same number of particles as that quantity of any other gas
- **B** occupies the same volume as one gram molecular weight of any other gas at any temperature
- **C** occupies 22.4 L at room temperature
- **D** depends on its vapour density
- **E** contains 6×10^{23} particles.

II.55 **The amount of a gas that dissolves in a liquid:**
- **A** will decrease if the temperature decreases
- **B** is independent of the nature of the gas
- **C** can be measured either by the Bunsen or Ostwald solubility coefficient
- **D** is governed by Henry's law
- **E** is independent of other gases that may be present.

II.56 Gas cylinders:
A are made of manganese steel to withstand high pressures
B the colour of the plastic ring around the neck denotes the year in which the cylinder was made
C the interval between cylinder testing is 2 years
D the actual maximum pressure which a cylinder can withstand is normally 65–70% above the working pressure
E on large, bull-nosed cylinders, instead of the pin-index system different screw threads are used for inflammable and non-inflammable gases.

II.57 In the SI system of measurement:
A the unit of time is the second
B the unit of length is defined using the wavelength of a particular emission of electromagnetic radiation
C the unit of temperature is approximately the same as the Centigrade degree
D the Newton is the derived unit of force
E the bel is a unit of energy.

II.58 Diffusion:
A Fick's law relates rate of diffusion to concentration gradient
B at tissue level, carbon dioxide equilibration takes place in less than 0.1 sec
C the diffusion rate of most volatile anaesthetics is approximately the same as carbon dioxide
D carbon monoxide and helium are used in the measurement of pulmonary diffusing capacity
E Graham's law directly relates rate of diffusion of a substance to its molecular size.

II.59 Safety – fires and explosions:
A in a stoichiometric mixture, the concentrations of vapour and oxidising agent are such that both are completely used up
B a stoichiometric mixture carries a maximal explosion risk
C the flammability limits of cyclopropane in oxygen are 30 – 60%
D nitrous oxide is an oxidising agent capable of supporting combustion
E the EEC definition of a zone of risk for the use of flammable gas mixtures is 25 cm from the apparatus.

II.60 Exponentials:
A in an exponential process, the rate of change of a quantity at any time is proportional to the quantity remaining at that time
B washout curves are exponential processes
C the total length of time taken by an exponential process is infinity
D after three half-lives of exponential decay, a quantity will have fallen to 1/4 of its initial value
E the time constant is the time at which the process would have been complete had the initial rate of change been maintained.

Paper II Answers

II.1 TTFFF

A The question does not qualify the acidosis. Remember that a primary respiratory acidosis would be caused by HYPOventilation.

C Reduced bicarbonate produces increased respiratory drive.

D Increased to increase H^+ production and excretion.

E H^+ excretion – acid urine.

II.2 TTTFF

C,D Are mutually exclusive.

E Vasoconstriction.

II.3 TTFFF

C Uric acid is a product of purine catabolism.

D Creatinine is synthsised from phosphocreatine.

E All amino-acids found in nature are L-forms.

II.4 TFTFF

A Peripheral pooling.

B Exercise increases cardiac output.

C Loss of the "muscle pump" reduces venous return.

D Cardiac output will increase to compensate for the shunt.

E Rapid infusion simulates venous return.

II.5 TFTFT

B,E The Q-T interval depends on the heart rate, the R-R interval is the reciprocal of the rate, the QRS is unaffected by the rate.

D There is no ejection during the phase of isovolumetric contraction.

II.6 FTTTF

A The membrane potential approaches the equilibrium potential for sodium (+60 mV).

B True, 0.4–1.0 msec.

C True, eg sympathetic fibres 2 msec.

E Refers to nodes of Ranvier, not salt!

II.7 TTTFT

D Increases glucagon secretion, driving potassium into cells.

E True; potassium passes into cells to maintain electrical neutrality.

II.8 TTTFF

Insulin is the main hormone of anabolism. It is extremely important and you should be clear about its many actions. Flow charts and diagrams are very helpful.

D It enhances uptake of ketones.

E Phosphorylation of glucose is controlled by other hormones, and the rapid phosphorylation maintains the concentration gradient for glucose across the cell membrane.

II.9 TTFTF

C Decreased effective ECF volume.

E A vasoconstrictor only in pharmacological concentrations.

II.10 TFFFF

B 17 to 26 days.

D Don't get muddled up with orthostatic proteinuria.

E The question doesn't say whether the increase is a systemic one or a local one distal to the site of occlusion. The answer is "false" anyway.

II.11 FTFTF

Good nutrition is essential for normal erythropoiesis and so a grossly deficient diet may affect red cell production in many ways. Cyanocobalamin (B12) and folate both play an essential, specific role, unlike vitamin C.

Vitamin E may be important in premature infants but certainly not in adults.

Valine is an essential amino-acid but that does not make it any more specifically involved with erythropoiesis than other essential amino-acids – its replacement by glutamic acid in sickle-cell anaemia is of genetic origin and is not caused by the non-availability of valine.

II.12 TFFFT

B   FDP's > 40.

C   Decreased due to consumption and subsequent lysis.

D   No – this is fibrinolysis, not haemolysis.

II.13 FFFFT

A   The glucose content is lower.

B   Lack of proteins means that buffering is less.

C   There are up to 3 lymphocytes per cubic millimetre.

D   It is a clear, colourless liquid.

II.14 FTTTF

It is beyond the scope of this book fully to explain the workings of the nephron – but it is very important. The counter-current system in particular needs clear thinking.

A   Ionic pumps are essential to the integrity of gradients in the kidney, but all the membranes are not uniformly permeable to water.

E   The loops of Henle are countercurrent multipliers, the vasa recta are countercurrent exchangers.

II.15 TTTFT

D   Renin release is unimportant in blood pressure maintenance with agents such as ether which are sympathetic stimulants, but IS important with sympathetic depressants such as halothane.

II.16   FFFFF

A   Barometric pressure falls and that reduces inspired and hence arterial oxygen, but the ventilatory response is not because of the reduced ambient pressure per se.

B   This occurs secondary to hyperventilation.

C   The hypoxia is relatively less because hyperventilation raises PaO_2 by reducing $PaCO_2$. It is the result of, not the reason for, hyperventilation.

D   This doesn't necessarily occur.

E   Hyperventilation may indeed occur secondary to this but not normally.

II.17   TFFFF

B   Rubbish, it's not a ratio!

C,D   Depends largely upon oxygen combined with haemoglobin.

E   20 vols%

II.18   FTFTF

A   'Diagnostic'' means that these symptoms could only be hypoxia, and that is obviously untrue.

B   An early sign and more reliable than hypertension.

C,D   Stimulation of the peripheral chemoreceptors causes increased ventilation and reflex hypertension. Eventually, if severe or protracted enough, there will be circulatory collapse.

E   Not always: not, for instance, in severe anaemia, carbon monoxide poisoning or cyanide poisoning.

II.19   TTFFT

You must know the oxyhaemoglobin dissociation curve. In an MCQ exam it is helpful to draw the curve on scrap paper before answering the question: the wording can be very confusing because the same condition can be presented in so many ways – for instance, **B** and **D** are both the effect of CO_2.

II.20   TTFFT

C   In elderly, though normal, subjects, some airways will be closed at FRC. Even in younger patients it is unlikely to be true: if "optimal" means unity then it is never true, if it means the best possible then it will remain so for a good range of lung expansion above FRC.

D   Compliance will be minimal at total lung capacity. It is maximal over a range of 1–2 litres above FRC.

II.21 FTTTF

    A   Most are not absorbed from the GI tract and there is no point in giving them orally for systemic infection. They CAN be given orally and neomycin is given to suppress intestinal bacteria, eg in preparation for some colonic surgery and also in severe liver failure.

    D   Because of foetal ototoxicity.

    E   Excretion is 100% renal.

II.22 FFTFF

    A   Usually unchanged but slight tachycardia possible.

    B   Vagal blockade produces tachycardia. Atropine can produce a centrally mediated bradycardia, though this is rarely marked.

    D   Increased cardiac output but rate unaffected.

    E   Acute increase then back to normal.

II.23 TFTTT

    A,B   Atropine reduces saturation by increasing physiological dead space.

    E   It reduces the integrity of the cardiac sphincter. This is one of the mechanisms by which atropine makes metoclopramide a less effective anti-emetic.

II.24 TFFTT

    A   It is non-selective: bronchial relaxation is beta–2.

    B   The vasodilatory antihypertensives are the ones likely to cause postural hypotension.

    C   Propranolol is particularly useful with high renin levels and actually reduces its production.

    D   By reducing cardiac contractility.

    E   It can block peripheral vasodilatation.

II.25 TTFTF

    C   Cardiacirritability is not increased and methoxamine can safely be used during anaesthesia with volatile agents.

    E   Is also often given intramuscularly for a more sustained effect.

II.26   FFTTF

The question implies "clinically useful" anticonvulsants.
B   Suxamethonium prevents the muscular manifestations only.
E   Lignocaine can be used in status epilepticus as a last resort; on the other hand its toxic effects are primarily on the CNS and include convulsions. The safe answer is "false"

II.27   FTTFF

A   Related to thiazides, but is a vasodilator.
D   It does, compare thiazide side effects.
E   It is.

II.28   FFTTF

B   Ganglion blockers, which may be used as intraoperative infusions, cause dilated pupils.
E   SNP infusions may cause a reflex tachycardia because of reflex sympathe– tic activity. The use of the infusion to produce hypotension may be thwarted by the tachycardia unless beta-blockers are given with the premedication or during the operation.

II.29   TTFTF

Pharmacological agents that stimulate the secretion of ADH are believed to be cholinergic agonists, PGE1 (although this inhibits its action on the kidney), and large doses of barbiturates. Morphine probably raises the threshold for secretion rather than actual release. Beta agonists cause antidiuresis; alpha agonists cause diuresis. One cannot know every effect of every drug. You may be lucky and pick up a mark for an occasional remembered connection but don't guess if you don't know. You should have known morphine and alcohol (which decreases secretion).
E   Probably has no effect either way.

II.30   TTTFF

A   Potency is an awkward word that means, strictly, the weight-for- weight effectiveness of a drug and says nothing about speed of action.
C,D   Muscular movements on induction are not necessarily epileptiform, but methohexitone does have convulsant activity in those prone to epilepsy.

II.31 FTTFF

A   50°C.
D   Attacks aluminium in vaporisers.
E   Decomposes unless stabilised with thymol.

II.32 FTFFT

A   Only free drug can be metabolised.
B   It will displace warfarin and increase the effect of a given
     dose.
C,D There is no connection.

II.33 FFFTT

A   10% and 20% solutions of mannitol are both hypertonic.
B   Though isosmolar, uptake of the sugar by the red cells
     soon renders 5% dextrose effectively hypotonic and the
     red cells lyse.
C   0.9M (molar) NaCl would be extremely hypertonic. A
     molar solution of NaCl contains 58.5 grams per litre.
     Remember that chemical and physiological "normality"
     are not the same. 0.9% NaCl is isotonic (9 grams/L).

II.34 TTTTT

A   True, increases proportion of ionised drug, therefore
     reducing reabsorption.
B   True, reduces ionised aspirin fraction and increases
     reabsorption.
D   Potassium excreted in preference to hydrogen ions.
E   Renal compensation for respiratory alkalosis.

II.35 TTTFT

A   True. Histamine itself is broken down by diamine oxidase
     (histaminase) and the resulting methyl-histamine is then
     metabolised by mono-amine oxidase.
D   The highest concentrations are in the liver.

II.36 TTFFT
- **C**   Not a feature of lignocaine toxicity.
- **D**   Bradycardia due to myocardial depression.

II.37 TFFTF
- **B**   Is antagonised, in vitro, by Ca^{2+}, and Ca^{2+} and Mg^{2+} usually have opposing actions.
- **D**   One third in urine, some in bile, some metabolised.
- **E**   Some, of course, will cross the placenta, but the actual quantity will be very small.

II.38 TTTTF
- **E**   Only stable for a matter of microseconds before hydrolysis leading to the re-formation of the enzyme and acetic acid.

II.39 FTFTT
- **A**   Certainly will!.
- **C**   No – would precipitate withdrawal symptoms.

II.40 TTFTF
- **A**   Peripheral vasoconstriction.
- **B**   Lactic acidosis.
- **C**   The interaction at the neuromuscular junction is with the aminoglycosides and some less commonly used antibiotics.
- **D**   Potentiation of action is because of displacement from protein binding sites.
- **E**   Chelation of tetracyclines, not chloramphenicol, by iron.

II.41 **TTFFT**

A   eg with a thermistor tipped flow-directed balloon-tipped catheter.

B   Much used in research, they are not so common clinically.

C   Stroke volume can be derived from a measurement of THORACIC impedance, although the impedance changes are much smaller than those caused by respiratory movements.

D   Will measure blood flow to the limb only.

II.42 **TTTTT**

E   True, potentials are microvolt, not millivolt.

II.43 **TTTTT**

All are suitable provided they can be converted into volatile compounds.

II.44 **TTFTT**

C   The other way around.

E   Applications such as infra-red CO_2 analysis and ultra-violet halothane analyser.

II.45 **TFTFT**

B   The closing volume is normally smaller than the FRC.

D   By a slow expiration, not a forced expiration. Also by total body plethysmography.

E   You should be able to draw, and to understand, the plot of tracer con— centration against volume obtained from this test.

II.46 TFTTT
- **B**   Student was a pseudonym used by the man who described the t distribution.

II.47 FFTTF
If you can derive this equation you will understand it better than if you merely learn it.
- **A**   The implication is that the pH DEPENDS on the ratio, not that it is constant.
- **B**   In vitro.
- **E**   See the Sigaard-Andersen nomogram.

II.48 FTFTT
- **A**   Inulin is freely filtered at the glomeruli (which is not the same as completely cleared). It is a useful biochemical tool because it is neither secreted or absorbed by the tubules.
- **C**   Blood urea is unaffected until glomerular filtration is considerably reduced.

II.49 TFFTF
- **A**   The normal red cell will lyse in saline more dilute than about 0.4–0.45%.
- **B**   290 mOsmol/L is correct, but it is mainly due to the ions: the oncotic pressure is mainly due to the proteins.
- **E**   Raoult's law: the depression of vapour pressure of a solvent is proportional to the molar concentration of the solute.

II.50 TFTTT
- **A**   Digital meters have no moving parts and therefore no inertia.
- **B**   That is usually the function of a filter, but it may not be the correct filter, or the signal and the unwanted noise may be of the same frequency and unseparable.

II.51   TFTTF

- **A**   The pressure will not be transmitted fully to the artery: as a rough guide the cuff should cover one third to one half of the upper arm from elbow to shoulder.
- **B**   Venous engorgement reduces accuracy.
- **C**   Only up to a point because the stimulus of the inflated cuff will raise the blood pressure and B.
- **E**   Systolic pressure agrees better. Correlation with diastolic pressure is complicated by differences in the phase of the Korotkov sounds deemed to correspond to the diastolic pressure.

II.52   TTTFT

- **D**   Lower potentials are used because the skin resistance is by-passed and the stimulus is nearer the nerve.

II.53   TTFTF

A rather awkward question because there is such a variety of ventilators. The true answers must be UNIVERSAL answers.

- **A**   Note that the tidal volume may be dependent on the frequency.
- **B**   The limit is usually the pressure relief valve on the ventilator which will be set at 50–60 cm H_2O or more.
- **D**   The upper airway pressure will be registered on the pressure gauge on the ventilator, provided there is no obstruction in the ventilator tubing or connections.
- **E**   It will depend on the particular ventilator.

II.54   TFFFT

- **A**   The temperature, pressure and volume are here irrelevant as it is a defined mass of gas.
- **B**   Must define pressure too.
- **C**   At STP: 0°C and 1 atmosphere (dry).
- **D**   The vapour density depends on the molecular weight, not the other way round.
- **E**   Actually 6.022×10^{23}, but 6 is near enough: consider the accuracy needed when answering any numerical question.

II.55   FFTTF

- **A**   Increases at lower temperatures.
- **B**   Defined by the solubility coefficient.
- **E**   Must be false: think of the situation of the chemical properties of other gases that might be present.

II.56   TFFTT
B   The coloured discs denote the year in which the cylinder was last tested.
C   The interval between cylinder testing is 5–10 years.
E   True: right-hand internal thread for air, helium and nitrogen; left-hand internal thread for hydrogen and inflammable gases.

II.57   TTTTF
B   The metre and Kr86.
C   The unit of temperature is the Kelvin.
D   Mass × acceleration = $m\ kg\ s^{-2}$
E   The Bel is a unit for describing power ratios. It is a logarithmic description, so a ratio of 10 times is 1 bel.

II.58   TTTTF
E   Graham's law states that the rate of diffusion of a gas is inversely proportional to the square root of its molecular weight.

II.59   TTFTT
C   Much wider: 2.5–60%.
D   True. Nitrous oxide rapidly breaks down if hot enough to produce a 33% oxygen mixture.

II.60   TTTFT
D   After three half-lives, the quantity is reduced to 1/8, ie 2 cubed.

Paper III Questions

III.1 Buffer mechanisms:
- **A** exist to allow time for respiratory compensation
- **B** quantitatively, the most important extracellular mechanism involves haemoglobin
- **C** in a chronic acidosis, ammonium excretion allows bicarbonate conservation and maintenance of buffering capacity
- **D** in the carbonic acid/bicarbonate system, the normal ratio of concentrations of unionised to ionised is 20 to 1
- **E** plasma proteins are a relatively unimportant buffer mechanism in man.

III.2 Alpha adrenergic stimulation produces:
- **A** vasodilation
- **B** tachycardia
- **C** uterine relaxation
- **D** a positive inotropic effect
- **E** intestinal relaxation.

III.3 Pyruvate:
- **A** is a 3-carbon carboxylic acid
- **B** is converted to phosphoenolpyruvate by pyruvate kinase
- **C** enters the carboxylic acid cycle after conversion to oxaloacetate by pyruvate carboxylase
- **D** is converted from alanine by an aminotransferase reaction
- **E** its main metabolite is via decarboxylation to acetyl coA.

III.4 The QRS deflection on the electrocardiogram is:
- **A** normally longer than 0.2 sec.
- **B** caused by ventricular repolarisation
- **C** prolonged in bundle branch block
- **D** associated with the phase of isovolumetric contraction
- **E** absent in complete block of atrio-ventricular conduction.

III.5 The coronary blood flow:
- **A** is about 250 ml per minute at rest
- **B** the oxygen uptake is about 40 ml per minute at rest
- **C** is altered directly by vagal activity
- **D** ceases in systole
- **E** shows autoregulation.

III.6   Synapses:

   A   in mammalian nerve, the synaptic cleft is 200 Angstrom units
   B   in the CNS are mainly in white matter
   C   only permit conduction in one direction
   D   are present in the sympathetic and parasympathetic ganglia
   E   are present in the dorsal root ganglia.

III.7   Calcium balance:

   A   vitamin D stimulates calcium reabsorption from gut, bones and renal tubules
   B   parathormone elevates serum calcium
   C   calcitonin reduces serum calcium
   D   calcium absorption is reduced by steroids
   E   calcium is excreted only in urine.

III.8   Angiotensin II:

   A   acts directly on vascular smooth muscle rather than via alpha receptors
   B   is formed in the lungs
   C   is an octapeptide
   D   manufacture from Angiotensin I is by the same enzyme that breaks down bradykinin
   E   is decreased when a subject stands after a period of sitting.

III.9   Antidiuretic hormone:

   A   acts throughout the body to conserve fluid
   B   induces smooth muscle constriction
   C   may produce coronary vasoconstriction
   D   acts via cyclic AMP
   E   induces phosphorylation of cell membranes, increasing permeability to water.

III.10 In exercise:

   A   oxygen consumption rises in relation to lactate production
   B   mixed venous oxygen tension decreases
   C   plasma antidiuretic hormone concentrations fall
   D   the number of patent capillaries in skeletal muscle increases
   E   systemic blood flow rises more rapidly than pulmonary blood flow.

III.11 In the blood:

    A basophils account for less than 0.5% of the total white count

    B megakaryocytes break up to form platelets

    C opsonisation facilitates phagocytosis by neutrophils

    D the majority of lymphocytes are of extramedullary origin

    E each red cell contains about 29 picograms of haemoglobin.

III.12 Causes of the anticoagulent effect of a massive blood transfusion includes:

    A deficient factor V and VIII

    B inactive platelets

    C microaggregates

    D cold

    E vitamin K availability.

III.13 The knee jerk:

    A is a monosynaptic reflex

    B arises from the spinal cord at T12

    C afferents are from the quadriceps tendon

    D is not controlled by higher centres

    E afferents come from the quadriceps muscle.

III.14 The concentration gradient in the renal medulla:

    A is generated in equal part by each nephron

    B is independent of urine flow

    C depends on active transport of sodium

    D urea maintains the high osmolality in the pyramids

    E can be maintained by aerobic or anaerobic metabolism.

III.15 Sympatho-adrenal activation:

    A may induce shunting of blood within the kidney

    B reduces proximal tubular reabsorption of certain ions

    C increases net filtration pressure within Bowman's capsule

    D increases renal blood flow

    E is prevented by dopamine therapy.

III.16 **The main features of acclimatisation to high altitude are:**
   A   an increase in oxygen carrying capacity
   B   an increase in respiratory minute volume
   C   an increase in cardiac output
   D   a compensatory decrease in heart rate
   E   redistribution of blood flow away from the pulmonary
       vascular bed.

III.17 **Breathing carbon monoxide even in small amounts is
dangerous because:**
   A   carbon monoxide has a great affinity for reduced
       haemoglobin
   B   blood can be completely saturated with carbon monoxide at
       a partial pressure of 0.66 kPa (5 mm Hg)
   C   when the whole of the available haemoglobin is saturated
       with carbon monoxide, no oxygen can be carried
   D   carboxyhaemoglobin dissociation is irreversible within 2
       hours
   E   carboxyhaemoglobin alters red cell shape leading to
       aggregation.

III.18 **Hypercapnia:**
   A   causes sweating
   B   increases parasympathetic activity
   C   at extremes, will depress ventilation
   D   has a direct inotropic action as well as its autonomic effects
   E   aids the uptake of oxygen in the lung.

III.19 **Stagnant hypoxia:**
   A   is caused by a sluggish peripheral circulation
   B   is associated with stagnant oxygen in the blood
   C   occurs when the mean pulmonary capillary diffusion
       constant is reduced
   D   is temperature dependent
   E   is dependent upon the haemoglobin concentration.

III.20 **Apart from that carried in simple solution, carbon dioxide is
carried in the blood:**
   A   in the red cells
   B   as carbonic acid, which is buffered
   C   in direct combination with oxyhaemoglobin
   D   as phosphate esters
   E   combined with plasma protein.

III.21 Erythromycin:
- **A** is a good alternative to penicillin in penicillin allergy
- **B** is well tolerated even in large doses
- **C** is used in Legionnaire's disease
- **D** causes cholestatic jaundice
- **E** the dose must not exceed 1G per day.

III.22 Noradrenaline depletion is produced by:
- **A** reserpine
- **B** phentolamine
- **C** pempidine
- **D** guanethidine
- **E** hydralazine.

III.23 Atropine:
- **A** inhibits sweating
- **B** crosses the placental barrier
- **C** possesses local anaesthetic effects
- **D** is totally metabolised in the liver
- **E** increases tone in the internal laryngeal muscles.

III.24 Propranolol:
- **A** decreases cardiac output
- **B** causes tachycardia
- **C** can cause bradycardia
- **D** suppresses secretion of renin
- **E** is useful in the treatment of heart failure.

III.25 Drugs which exert an autonomic ganglion blocking effect include:
- **A** decamethonium
- **B** barbiturates
- **C** atropine
- **D** trimetaphan
- **E** phentolamine.

III.26 Midazolam:

    A is water soluble

    B accumulates in body fat

    C is rarely associated with venous thrombosis

    D should not be given a second time within two weeks

    E may induce epileptiform EEG changes.

III.27 A metabolic alkalosis inhibits the diuretic action of:

    A spironolactone

    B chlorothiazide

    C acetazolamide

    D mersalyl

    E frusemide.

III.28 Sodium nitroprusside;

    A affects both resistance and capacitance vessels

    B reduces renal blood flow

    C is metabolised to ferrocyanide

    D should be made up for infusion in 5% dextrose

    E is contra-indicated in phaeochromocytoma.

III.29 The hypoglycaemic effect of the sulphonylureas is reduced by:

    A propranolol

    B phenylbutazone

    C intravenous calcium gluconate

    D the oral contraceptives

    E bendrofluazide.

III.30 For use, a new intravenous induction agent must:

    A be water soluble

    B have a pH of 7.4

    C cross the blood-brain barrier

    D be stable in solution

    E be completely broken down in the body within one hour.

III.31 Ketamine:

    A is a potent analgesic

    B is rapidly metabolised in the liver

    C releases noradrenaline

    D produces muscular relaxation

    E does not depress the cardiovascular system.

III.32 Competitive antagonism:

    A usually refers to competition with enzymes at the site of action of the drug

    B is shown by a rightward shift of the dose-response curve

    C is true of the competition of cyanides and nitrites for the cytochrome system

    D is true of beta-adrenergic blockers and sympathomimetic amines

    E is only possible if the receptors are fully occupied.

III.33 Morphine is metabolised by:

    A conjugation with a glucuronide

    B mono-amine oxidase

    C acetylation

    D N-dealkylation

    E hydrolysis.

III.34 Antihistaminic activity is associated with:

    A promethazine

    B ranitidine

    C cyclizine

    D mepyramine

    E chlorpheniramine.

III.35 Carbonic anhydrase:

    A catalyses the formation of carbonic acid from carbon dioxide

    B is present in greater quantities in the gastric oxyntic cells than in the red blood cells

    C increases the production of aqueous humour

    D inhibitors affect renal tubular function

    E inhibitors produce respiratory depression.

III.36 Procaine:

A   is an amide
B   should not be used with sulphonamides
C   antagonises the metabolism of propanidid
D   may produce central stimulation
E   produces mild ganglionic blockade.

III.37 These drugs are inactivated by plasma cholinesterase:

A   propanidid
B   suxamethonium
C   procaine
D   decamethonium
E   gallamine.

III.38 Non-depolarising neuromuscular blocking drugs:

A   are potentiated by cyclopropane
B   are potentiated more by ether than by methoxyflurane
C   are potentiated by intraperitoneal kanamycin
D   may be potentiated in patients with multiple neurofibromatosis
E   are potentiated in hyperkalaemia.

III.39 Pethidine:

A   increases cerebrospinal fluid pressure
B   is a local analgesic
C   produces vasoconstriction
D   does not produce constipation
E   has an anticholinergic action.

III.40 The following have interactions likely to be of clinical importance:

A   lithium carbonate and hyponatraemia
B   prednisolone and carbenoxolone
C   insulin and phenoxybenzamine
D   dapsone and probenecid
E   labetolol and ranitidine.

III.41 When measuring central venous pressure:

A a catheter should not be advanced further than 20 cm in any patient

B the diameter of the catheter should not exceed 0.25 mm

C the subclavian route is useful

D the zero point should be taken from the sternal angle even when the patient is sitting up

E a dependent loop of tubing should be avoided to prevent back flow of blood into the catheter.

III.42 Biological potentials:

A the potentials involved in the EEG are in the region of 50 microvolts

B the beta waves of the EEG occur in the 15–60 Hz range

C the alpha waves of the EEG occur in the 70–100 Hz range

D because of the small potentials involved, accidental electrocution is not a risk when measuring the EEG

E the EMG is unlikely to interfere with the EEG because of the difference in electrical potentials involved.

III.43 In a fit 30 year old male:

A the alveolar ventilation at rest is 4.2 L/min

B the maximum voluntary ventilation is 125 – 170 L/min

C the functional residual capacity is 1.2 L

D at maximum inspiration, intrapleural pressure falls to −30 cm water

E the total area available for gas exchange is approximately 20 m^2.

III.44 Infra-red gas analysers measure:

A carbon monoxide

B carbon dioxide

C nitrous oxide

D ether

E halothane.

III.45 Which of the following statements are true:

A carbon monoxide is used in the measurement of functional residual capacity

B the measurement of pulmonary gas transfer factor necessitates the use of an inert gas such as helium

C the normal FEV1/FVC ratio should be in excess of 75% in a 50 year old man

D 0.3 ml oxygen per 100 ml blood are dissolved when breathing room air and with a haemoglobin of 15 gm/dl

E approximately 72% of the blood volume is contained within the normal venous circulation.

III.46 A non-parametric test:

A   can apply to samples that are not distributed normally
B   can be used on small samples
C   are generally mathematically easier than parametric tests
D   imply that the variable cannot be measured accurately
E   an example is the Wilcoxon matched pairs signed rank test.

III.47 In an uncompensated respiratory alkalosis:

A   the patient will be hypoventilating
B   the base excess may exceed 10 mmol/L
C   the pHa may be 7.65 or above
D   the concentration of ionised calcium in the plasma is decreased.
E   the patient may show signs of tetanus.

III.48 The extracellular fluid:

A   is approximately 20% of the body weight in the average adult male
B   does not include the cerebrospinal fluid
C   the volume can be measured directly by dilution techniques
D   the volume can be measured using deuterium oxide
E   contains more chloride than bicarbonate.

III.49 The following cause movement of water and solute between compartments in vivo:

A   solvent drag
B   filtration
C   osmosis
D   pinocytosis
E   diffusion.

III.50 Electromagnetic radiation:

A   includes visible light
B   infra-red radiation only occurs from objects that are hotter than the environment
C   Stefan's law defines the heat radiated from a black body and includes a term of the fourth power of the absolute temperature of the body
D   obeys the inverse square law
E   includes ultrasound.

III.51 An oscillotonometer:
  A relies on the intrinsic oscillatory properties of aneroids
  B must be read when the leak is closed
  C can be used as an ordinary blood pressure cuff by
     auscultation or palpation
  D is inaccurate at altitude
  E performs best if the patient is vasoconstricted.

III.52 Oscilloscopes:
  A the electron beam is deflected in the X axis by applying a
     "saw-tooth" potential to the deflecting plates
  B the ECG signal deflects the beam in the Y axis
  C under normal circumstances, the calibration is 1 mV to
     produce a 1 mm deflection
  D the low inertia of the electron beam limits the frequency
     response of the instrument
  E in a memory oscilloscope, the incoming signal is divided
     into discrete blocks which are displayed digitally.

**III.53 If a ventilator is a minute volume divider and a pressure
generator:**
  A the tidal volume will fall as the resistance rises
  B the ventilatory frequency is a function of the tidal volume
  C increasing the minute volume increases the tidal volume
     and the inspiratory flow rate
  D increasing the pressure increases the inspiratory flow rate
  E tidal volume may fall if the compliance rises.

**III.54 The following need to be known to calculate the volume of
vapour obtained at STP from the complete evaporation of a
liquid:**
  A the saturated vapour pressure of the liquid
  B Avogadro's number
  C the liquid density
  D the molecular weight
  E the volume of liquid.

III.55 When a liquid boils:
  A its vapour pressure is 1 atmosphere (101 kPa)
  B its latent heat of vaporisation is zero
  C bubbles of vapour form on irregularities in the container
  D the temperature of the liquid cannot exceed the boiling point
  E it will contain little or no dissolved gas.

III.56 In the measurement of carbon dioxide:

A   the Lloyd-Haldane apparatus can measure in the gas or liquid phase

B   infra-red absorption can be used

C CO_2 absorbs light at a wavelength of 430 nM

D   carbon monoxide may interfere

E   cannot be distinguished from nitrous oxide with a mass spectrometer.

III.57 The following statements are true:

A   the maximum total whole body dose of radioactivity to a person working with radiation is 4 rems per calendar month

B   the half life of iodine–131 is 8 days

C   the SI unit of visible light wavelength is the Angstrom

D   1 ml of blood will dissolve 0.0021 ml of oxygen at 37°C and a PO_2 of 93 kPa (700 mm Hg)

E   the peak voltage of the AC supply in the UK is 325 V.

III.58 Osmosis:

A   osmolarity refers to the number of mosmoles per litre of water

B   osmolality refers to the number of mosmoles per litre of a specific solvent

C   the depression of freezing point of a solution is inversely proportional to its osmolality

D   Raoult's law states that the depression or lowering of vapour pressure of a solvent is proportional to the molar concentration of the solute

E   osmometers can also work on the principle of vapour pressure depression.

III.59 Safety – fires and explosions:

A   the flammability limits of ether in oxygen are 2 to 82%

B   the stoichiometric concentration of ether in oxygen is 14%

C   ethyl chloride vapour is flammable

D   halothane is non-inflammable

E   the stoichiometric concentration of ethyl alcohol skin preparation in air is 70%.

III.60 The sine function:

A   is the pattern of alternating current (AC)

B   describes the motion of a freely-moving pendulum

C   has a maximal value of 1 and a minimum of 0

D   is a hyperbolic function

E   is the natural logarithm of the cosine.

Paper III Answers

III.1 FTTFF

- **A** For renal compensation.
- **D** Correct ratio but wrong way round. Ionised:unionised = 20:1.
- **E** Quantitatively important in blood.

III.2 TFFFT

- **B** Reflex bradycardia, but no direct effect.
- **C** Assuming that it is pregnant uterine tone, noradrenaline increases it.
- **D** No inotropic effect.
- **E** True, but gastrointestinal sphincteric tone is increased.

III.3 TFTTT

- **A** $CH_3.CO.COOH$
- **B** It is an irreversible reaction in the other direction.
- **C** This is true, but acetyl coenzyme-A is the more important route (**E**).

III.4 FFTTF

- **A** $0.08 - 0.10$ sec.
- **B** The QRS is ventricular DEpolarisation, the T wave is REpolarisation.
- **C** It is particularly prolonged in left bundle branch block.
- **D** This phase ends when the tricuspid and mitral valves open. There is no direct causative relation between the QRS and this phase, but they do occur at the same time.
- **E** Complexes will be abnormal, but absence would cause Stokes-Adams attacks or death.

III.5 TTFFT

- **C** The question says "directly" but the vagus alters coronary blood flow indirectly via its negative inotropic effect.
- **D** Two thirds during diastole; one third during systole. However there is no subendocardial flow during systole.

III.6   TFTTT

   B   In the grey matter of the CNS.

III.7   TTTTF

   D   Steroids depress vitamin D stimulation of calcium
          absorption.
   E   Mainly secreted into the gut.

III.8   TTTTF

   B   70% of Angiotensin I is converted to Angiotensin II during
          a single passage through the lung. This conversion also
          occurs in other tissues.
   D   Peptidyl dipeptidase. Captopril, used in the treatment of
          hypertension, inhibits this enzyme and thus blocks the
          synthesis of both the most active vasoconstrictor known
          (Ang II) and the breakdown of most potent vasodilator
          known (bradykinin).

III.9   TTTTT

III.10   FTFTF

   A   Both rise but not in relation to each other, one is aerobic,
          the other anaerobic
   C   Rise.
   E   Impossible!

III.11 TFTTT
- **A**   0.4%
- **B**   This is true, but occurs in the marrow.
- **C**   Opsonins coat bacteria and render them more attractive to the phagocytes.
- **D**   The majority are formed in the lymph nodes, thymus and spleen.

III.12 TTTFF
- **D**   Cold normally has no effect, but rarely may cause agglutination.
- **E**   Vitamin K is stored over a long time and acute deficiency does not occur.

III.13 TFFTT
- **A**   It is an example of the stretch reflex, the only monosynaptic reflex.
- **B**   L 3–4.
- **C**   The afferents are the muscle spindles within the muscle. The receptors in the tendons are the Golgi tendon organs that subserve the inverse stretch reflex, a bi-synaptic reflex.
- **D**   It is not controlled by the higher centres, but it can be modified by them.

III.14 FFTTF
- **A**   Not all the loops are of equal length.
- **B**   Very high flow can wash solutes out of the medulla.
- **C,E**   As it depends on active sodium transport, it must rely on aerobic metabolism.

III.15 TTTTF
- **E**   Only produces localised vasodilation, by direct stimulation of dopaminergic receptors.

III.16 TTTFF

A   Polycythaemia.
C   True, but unimportant by comparison with changes in respiration.
D   Tachycardia.

III.17 TTTFF

D   Carbon monoxide is reversible as soon as higher concentrations of oxygen are given.
E   No – this is sickle cell disease, haemoglobin S.

III.18 TTTFF

B   The parasympathetic activity is present but overshadowed by concurrent sympathetic activity.
D CO_2 itself is a negative inotrope. Its effects via SNS reflexes and catecholamine secretion are positively inotropic.
E   The dissociation curve moves to the right, oxygen affinity is decreased and thus it is release in the tissues that is facilitated.

III.19 TFFTT

B   Stagnation refers to the blood.
C   Pulmonary gas transfer is not involved – if this constant exists at all!
E   Haemoglobin concentration determines oxygen content.

III.20 TTFFF

C   With reduced haemoglobin.

Rubbish!

III.21 TFTTF

B   Not toxic, but likely to cause nausea, vomiting and diarrhoea.

D   This is probably an allergic type of reaction.

E   250–500 mgm every 6 hours or up to 4G daily in severe infections.

III.22 TFFTF

B   Alpha adrenergic blocker.

C   Ganglion blocker.

D   True in spleen, heart and blood vessels.

E   Direct acting vasodilator.

III.23 TTTFF

D   Enzyme hydrolysis occurs both in the liver and in other tissues.

E   Has no effect.

III.24 TFTTF

D   It is particularly useful in hypertension in which there are high renin levels.

E   It is a negative inotrope and could make heart failure worse. It could help failure caused by a supraventricular tachycardia, but the sensible answer to this option is "false".

III.25 TTTTF

A   Similar structure to acetylcholine.

B,C Probably act on pre-ganglionic nerve endings, changing properties necessary for normal transmission.

D   Competitive ganglion blocker.

E   Alpha adrenergic blocker.

III.26 TTTFF
- **D** No evidence.
- **E** The benzodiazepines are anti-convulsants.

III.27 FFFTF
- **A** Aldosterone antagonist.
- **C** A carbonic anhydrase inhibitor used to treat metabolic alkalosis.
- **D** True: excess loss of chloride over bicarbonate produces metabolic alkalosis and mercurous ion is not converted to the active mercuric form.
- **E** Loop diuretic – unaffected.

III.28 TFFTF
- **B** In the hypotension of hypovolaemia renal blood flow is compromised by vasoconstriction; the hypotension produced by properly used SNP is associated with vasodilatation and renal blood flow is not compromised.
- **C** In the treatment of CN^- poisoning: CN^- + thiosulphate = thiocyanate. Ferrocyanide is not formed at all, either as a result of body metabolism or therapeutic intervention.

III.29 FFFTT
Always be wary if a diabetic on oral hypoglycaemics is on multiple therapy. The hypoglycaemic effect may be enhanced by, amongst others, beta-blockers **(A)** and agents that are strongly protein-bound **(B)**. Beta-blockers can also mask the symptoms and signs of hypoglycaemia.
- **C** A red herring: calcium has no known important effect either way.

III.30 FFTTF
The question does not say "the ideal agent" but just "a new agent."

III.31 TTTFT

D   Tends to produce hypertonus.

III.32 FTFTF

A   No: to specific receptors, usually components of cell membranes.

B   Non-competitive antagonism will also cause this at low drug concentrations.

C CN^- causes irreversible chelation of the metallic moiety of cytochrome oxidase. Nitrites cause the formation of methaemoglobin and the Fe^{3+} chelates the CN^-.

III.33 TFFTF

The basic principle in the metabolism of most drugs is to make them more water-soluble so that they can be excreted in the urine. All these mechanisms **(A-E)** have this function, but only **A** and **E** apply to morphine.

III.34 TTTTT

III.35 TTTTF

B   True, there are 5–6 times as much enzyme present in gastric cells.

D   True, although almost 99% inhibition must be present for this to be significant.

E   Inhibition leads to carbon dioxide accumulation and therefore respiratory stimulation.

III.36 FTTTT

    A   Is an ester.

    B   True, procaine is metabolised to para-amino benzoic acid which inhibits the action of sulphonamides.

    C   Both are hydrolysed by plasma cholinesterase.

III.37 TTTFF

    E   Renal excretion.

III.38 TTTTF

    E   Hyperkalaemia may be precipitated by suxamethonium but does not alter the response to non-depolarisers.

III.39 TTFTT

    C   Mild vasodilation and quinidine-like effect leading to a fall in blood pressure.

III.40 TTFTF

    A   Increased risk of lithium toxicity.

    B   Potassium loss.

    C   No: the interaction is with beta blockers.

    D   Excretion of dapsone is reduced because tubular secretion is slowed and so side-effects increase. This is an important principle, but this particular interaction is very small print for the anaesthetist.

    E   Cimetidine, but not ranitidine, decreases metabolism of beta-blockers.

III.41 FFTFF
- A   eg a long catheter from the antecubital fossa.
- B   Read carefully: a quarter of a millimetre!
- D   You should be able to discuss the details of the measurement of the CVP and the merits and accuracy of the various sites taken as zero.
- E   There SHOULD be a loop to prevent air embolus.

III.42 TTFFF
- C   Too large, 7–10 Hz range, smaller the beta waves.
- D   The current is from OUTSIDE due to faulty apparatus and NOT from INSIDE.
- E   The potentials overlap considerably – EMG=10–80 microvolts.

III.43 TTFTF
- C   This value is for residual volume – FRC is 2.2 L.
- E   Much more : 70 m^2.

III.44 TTTTT

III.45 FFTTT
- A,B Helium dilution is used to measure the FRC, carbon monoxide to estimate the transfer factor.

III.46 TTTFT

    D   Non-parametric tests are generally concerned with whether something occurred or not, or into what class division an observation can be put. There is no implication about the accuracy of the observed variable.

III.47 FFTTF

    A   By definition, a respiratory alkalosis is caused by hyperventilation.

    B   If uncompensated, the base excess (metabolic component) will be zero.

    E   You are unlikely to meet a question like this in the actual exam; it is here merely to stress the importance of reading the question – it should, of course, read "tetany" and the answer would then be "true".

III.48 TFTFT

    B   Strictly the CSF is part of the ECF although equilibration between the CSF and the rest of the ECF is slow.

    D   Not possible because D_2O is freely diffusible throughout the total body water (and can be used as an indicator to measure it).

III.49 TTTT

III.50 TFTTF

    B   There may not be net heat transfer but that does not mean that there isn't infra-red radiation.

    D   Ultrasound is, as the name implies, sound energy.

III.51 FTTFF

A   Aneroids have no more intrinsic oscillatory properties than any other closed box.

B   The needle will oscillate if the leak is open.

D   Unaffected by altitude: both aneroids are connected ultimately to the atmosphere.

E   Performs best when there is moderate hypotension and peripheral vaso– dilatation.

III.52 TTFFT

C   1 mV produces a 1 cm deflection.

D   The low inertia allows, not prevents, a very high frequency response.

III.53 FTFTF

An example would be the Manley ventilator. Remember, because there is such a variety of different ventilators, the true answers must be universal.

A   Not necessarily unless the inspiratory period is short or the resistance very high.

C   It will increase the tidal volume but not the flow rate unless the pressure is altered as well **(D)**.

E   Tidal volume may fall if compliance FALLS.

III.54 FFTTT

A   The SVP will tell something of the RATE of evaporation but not the total.

B   The number of particles in a mole of a substance (6.022 × 10^{23}.

III.55 FFTFT

A   The VP will equal the ambient pressure, which may be 101 kPa but depends on altitude and prevailing conditions.

B   The energy for vaporisation has to be supplied for the liquid to keep boiling. Only at the critical temperture does LH(vap) = 0.

C   As well as on particles in the liquid.

D   Superheated water, for instance.

III.56 FTTFF

A   Only in the gas phase.
D   Nitrous oxide may interfere.
E CO_2 and N_2O have the same mass number (44) but the gases can be separated by identification of fragments produced by ionisation (eg NO).

III.57 TTFFT

A   This is "true", but you can't know everything.
C   The nanometer (10^{-9} metres) = 10 Angstrom units (10^{-8} centimetres).
D   The figures here can be confusing, so try remembering one set of values and then working from that: under normal conditions (37°C, PaO_2=100 mm Hg) 100 ml of blood contains 20 ml of oxygen (19.7 ml as oxyhaemoglobin and 0.3 ml dissolved). The correct figure here should be 0.02 mls.
E   The quoted voltage (240) is RMS (root mean square).

III.58 FFFTT

A   Milliosmoles per litre of solvent involved.
B   Milliosmoles per kilogram of solvent.
C   Directly proportional.

III.59 TTTFF

D   Careful – halothane is only non-flammable in anaesthetic concentrations, the absolute limits of flammability are higher.
E   Only 6% and therefore very close to that achieved clinically.

III.60 TTFFF

C   A sine wave is symmetrical around a mean of zero, maximum is +1 and minimum is −1.
D   It is what it is – a sine function. It is an example of a trigonometric function.
E   The inverse of the cosine.

Paper IV   Questions

IV.1 Bicarbonate:

    A is produced in the renal tubular cell under the influence of carbonic anhydrase

    B concentration in cells is 5 mmol/L

    C concentration in plasma is 25 mmol/L

    D the bicarbonate space is approximately 10 litres in a 70 kg man

    E concentrations rise in potassium depletion.

IV.2 Some end products of protein metabolism in man include:

    A glycine

    B uric acid

    C urea

    D ammonia

    E sulphates.

IV.3 In cell metabolism:

    A the Kreb's cycle can operate for a limited time anaerobically

    B 1 molecule of glucose will yield 38 molecules of ATP

    C the aerobic oxidation of glucose is 100% efficient

    D the components of the Kreb's cycle are supplied entirely from carbohydrate metabolism

    E the RQ is higher for carbohydrates than fats because extra oxygen is needed to burn carbohydrate.

IV.4 On rising from the supine to the upright position:

    A the total peripheral resistance increases

    B cerebral blood flow falls

    C the heart rate increases

    D output of aldosterone and renin increases

    E changes may be more marked if there is hypovolaemia

IV.5 Concerning the cardiac output in man:

    A myocardial contractility is increased by adrenergic stimulation

    B cardiac index decreases with increasing age

    C myocardial contractility is increased in hypoxia

    D a rise in ventricular filling pressure increases stroke volume

    E cardiac output decreases in fever.

IV.6   Which of the following are true:

A   vertebrate myelinated nerve fibres are between 1 and 20 microns in diameter

B   when a nerve impulse reaches the muscle 'end-plate' electrical transmission occurs

C   5-hydroxytryptamine is one of the neurotransmitters at the skeletal neuromuscular junction

D   the motor neurones running to intrafusal fibres are gamma-motor fibres

E   fusimotor nerves are afferent only.

IV.7   Phosphate balance:

A   50% of total body phosphate is in bone

B   normal plasma phosphate is 0.8–1.4 mmol/L

C   serum phosphate levels are decreased by parathormone

D   phosphate is important in intracellular buffering systems

E   phosphate is important in the formation of high energy nucleotides.

IV.8   The following hormones have their action via adenylate cyclase:

A   parathyroid hormone

B   angiotensin

C   growth hormone

D   glucagon

E   alpha and beta adrenergic actions of catecholamines.

IV.9   Endorphins:

A   are short chain peptides

B   there is a homogeneous population of receptors for them

C   are present in the brain but not the spinal cord

D   concentrations are decreased by exercise

E   may be antagonised by naloxone.

IV.10 The sodium pump:

A   maintains the potential difference across cell membranes

B   involves adenyl cyclase activation

C   also affects intracellular potassium concentrations

D   involves different mechanisms in different cells

E   maintains an intracellular sodium concentration of 5–10 mmol/L

IV.11 Erythropoietin:

    A   production is increased in hypoxia

    B   renal erythropoietic factor is produced in the juxta-glomerular cells

* **C**   erythropoietin is still produced in nephrectomised man

    D   erythropoietin production is inhibited by steroids

    E   renal erythropoietic factor acts upon a plasma globulin to produce erythropoietin.

IV.12 Pathological bleeding due to excessive fibrinolysis is associated with:

    A   reduced fibrinogen

    B   elevated fibrin degradation products

    C   reduced plasminogen

    D   a PTT less than 30 seconds

    E   euglobulin clot lysis time greater than 2 hours.

IV.13 The velocity of impulse propagation along a nerve:

    A   increases with pressure on the nerve

    B   increases in metabolic acidosis

    C   increases when the serum potassium is low

    D   is greater in motor than in sensory nerves

    E   increases with the frequency of stimulation.

IV.14 Antidiuretic hormone:

    A   is a polypeptide

    B   will be secreted in response to an increase in the tonicity of extracellular fluid

    C   acts on the proximal and distal convoluted tubules altering the permeability to water

    D   acts via adenyl cyclase

    E   is released following activity of the osmoreceptors in the supraoptic nucleus.

IV.15 The effects of cortisol within the kidney are:

    A   increased free water clearance

    B   decreased sodium reabsorption

    C   increased glomerular filtration rate

    D   decreased water permeability of the collecting duct

    E   decreased renal molecular threshold.

IV.16 Physiologicaldead space:
- A   includes the anatomical dead space
- B   is unchanged over a two-fold range of tidal volume
- C   accounts for the difference in composition between "ideal" alveolar gas and mixed expired gas
- D   changes with posture
- E   is diffusion limited.

IV.17 The ability of the lungs to produce instantaneous gas exchange between air and pulmonary blood occurs because:
- A   the pulmonary capillaries perfuse about 70 square meters of alveolar tissue
- B   pulmonary capillaries are only 8 microns in diameter
- C   the alveolar capillary membrane is only two cells thick
- D   in alveoli, blood flows in one direction and gas in the other
- E   the alveolar-capillary membrane contains pores, 20 angstroms in diameter.

IV.18 Hypocapnia:
- A   raises the threshold to pain
- B   may cause clouding of consciousness
- C   causes vasoconstriction
- D   reduces intracerebral pressure by reducing the output of cerebrospinal fluid
- E   lowers plasma sodium.

IV.19 The saturation of arterial blood with oxygen depends on:
- A   alveolar oxygen tension
- B   haemoglobin content
- C   cardiac output
- D   arterial carbon dioxide tension
- E   arterial hydrogen ion concentration.

IV.20 Intrapleural pressure:
- A   is sub-atmospheric in normal quiet breathing
- B   may reach −30 mm Hg with increased inspiratory effort
- C   can be measured with an intragastric balloon
- D   is higher at the base than the apex when upright
- E   cannot rise above atmospheric pressure because the alveoli are open to the atmosphere.

IV.21 Cell wall synthesis is the primary site of action of:

  A chloramphenicol
  B penicillin
  C sulphonamides
  D tetracycline
  E aminoglycosides.

IV.22 Propranolol:

  A increases coronary blood flow
  B makes hay fever worse
  C alters glucose tolerance
  D increases blood pressure
  E reduces intracranial pressure.

IV.23 Hyoscine:

  A is a central nervous system depressant
  B reduces the intensity of opiate induced analgesia
  C is a respiratory depressant
  D induces bronchoconstriction
  E reduces motion sickness.

IV.24 In the treatment of paroxysmal ventricular tachycardia the following drugs are indicated:

  A digoxin
  B lignocaine
  C disopyramide
  D quinidine
  E verapamil.

IV.25 Guanethidine:

  A prevents noradrenaline release from nerve terminals
  B initially produces hypertension
  C guanethidine uptake into noradrenaline stores is prevented by amphetamine
  D residual effects can last for up to 3 days after stopping treatment
  E does not effect the parasympathetic system.

IV.26 Central sedation can be directly reversed by clinical doses of:

A   naloxone
B   physostigmine
C   doxapram
D   methylphenidate
E   nikethamide.

IV.27 Side effects of thiazide diuretics include:

A   reduced peripheral vascular tone
B   gout
C   potentiation of diabetes insipidus
D   pancreatitis
E   hyperkalaemia.

IV.28 Intralipid:

A   must be given through a central vein
B   may cause pyrexia and palpitations
C   it is safe to add drugs to the infusion bottle
D   the 10% solution is nearly isotonic
E   the 20% solution contains 8400 MJ/L(2000kcal/L).

IV.29 The barbiturates:

A   are a family of compounds derived from malonic and uric acids
B   become useful induction agents as their fat solubilities increase
C   were first used as induction agents in the first World War
D   become convulsant with N-substitution
E   show structural similarities with the butyrophenones.

IV.30 Diethyl ether:

A   is a safe anaesthetic agent for a Caesarian section
B   potentiates the action of non-depolarising muscle relaxants
C   is an irritant of the upper respiratory tract
D   is partially excreted through the skin
E   has an MAC of 1.9% in air.

IV.31 Isoflurane:

A   is a halogenated hydrocarbon that is a structural isomer of enflurane
B   is metabolised very little in humans
C   is a respiratory depressant
D   has a relatively high solubility in blood
E   causes less depression of blood pressure than does halothane.

IV.32 The binding of a drug to plasma proteins:

A   prolongs its biological half-life
B   is markedly different in arterial and venous blood
C   is only of importance to albumin
D   prevents rapid renal glomerular filtration of the drug
E   prevents renal tubular secretion of the drug.

IV.33 The following drugs will cross the normal blood-brain barrier:

A   streptomycin
B   sulphadimidine
C   penicillin
D   tubocurarine
E   diazepam.

IV.34 Bronchodilation occurs with

A   cyclopropane
B   trichloroethylene
C   halothane
D   diethyl ether
E   nitrous oxide.

IV.35 Proteinase inhibitors include

A   streptokinase
B   tranexamic acid
C   plasmin
D   aprotinin
E   epsilon amino caproic acid.

IV.36 Vasodilation by a direct effect is caused by

- A bupivacaine
- B cocaine
- C procaine
- D lignocaine
- E cinchocaine.

IV.37 The following drugs prolong the effect of suxamethonium:

- A atropine
- B propanidid
- C tacrine
- D lignocaine
- E ecothiopate.

IV.38 Opioid narcotics:

- A are all obtained by refining extracts of the opium poppy
- B their action is mainly non-specific on the reticular activating system
- C should only be given with caution to patients with hepatic dysfunction
- D are inactive by mouth
- E their effects are augmented by butryophenones.

IV.39 Pethidine:

- A produces mydriasis
- B has antihistaminic properties
- C has a quinidine-like myocardial depressant effect
- D is compatible with thiopentone in vitro
- E relieves ureteric colic.

IV.40 The following pairs of drugs can confidently be used safely together:

- A chlormethiazole and bishydroxycoumarin
- B halothane and succinylcholine
- C alpha-methyldopa and pargyline
- D phenobarbitone and penicillin
- E pancuronium and cefuroxime.

IV.41 **A sample of blood for gas analysis:**
- **A** should be taken in a glass syringe
- **B** should be withdrawn slowly to prevent gas coming out of the sample
- **C** should be stored at body temperature until analysis
- **D** should be withdrawn and then mixed with heparin
- **E** the heparin should contain at least 125,000 IU per ml.

IV.42 **Concerning blood pressure measurement:**
- **A** the width of the occluding cuff should be 20% greater than the diameter of the arm
- **B** too narrow a cuff will produce artificially reduced measurements of blood pressure
- **C** the Korotkoff sounds have five phases
- **D** in the Doppler method of detection, blood flow causes Doppler frequency shift
- **E** with an automatic cuff system (eg the Dinamap) pressure oscillations are sensed in the cuff commencing at systolic pressure and increasing until mean pressure is reached.

IV.43 **Dead space:**
- **A** anatomical dead space is approximately 2 ml/kg
- **B** physiological dead space is the total dead space minus the anatomical dead space
- **C** total dead space may be measured by single breath nitrogen washout
- **D** Bohr's equation for the calculation of total dead space requires the measurement of expired and alveolar PCO_2
- **E** in Bohr's equation the inspired PCO_2 can be ignored for clinical purposes.

IV.44 **Spectrophotometric ultra-violet analysers:**
- **A** are used for halothane since it absorbs ultra-violet radiation
- **B** are insensitive to carbon dioxide
- **C** are sensitive to nitrous oxide
- **D** use a mercury vapour discharge lamp to produce ultra-violet light at 2,357 Angstroms
- **E** are used in the estimation of barbiturates, eg thiopentone.

IV.45 **An end-tidal sample of expired air:**
- **A** has a carbon dioxide content of approximately 4.5%
- **B** is obtained by exhaling deeply into a gas sampling tube
- **C** is obtained by breathing into one end of an open tube 25mm in diameter and 1.5 metres long, and sampling from the other end
- **D** will have equilibrated with the pCO_2 of systemic arterial blood
- **E** is only of clinical use if obtained at the end of a forced expiration.

IV.46 In the interpretation of statistics:

    A paired tests are more powerful than unpaired tests

    B the confidence limits are usually taken to be an estimate of the 95% probability of the actual value of an observed variable or of the mean of a number of observations

    C the standard error of the mean is the confidence limit of the mean of a number of observations

    D the F test compares variances

    E the sample means from a population will be normally distributed.

IV.47 Hydrogen ions and ionisation:

    A a litre of pure water contains 10^{-7} grams of H^+ ions

    B pK varies with temperature

    C pH will be directly proportional to the log of the carbon dioxide tension

    D the acidity of a solution depends on the hydrogen ion activity, which is not necessarily equal to the concentration

    E a change of 1 pH unit means a one hundred fold change in hydrogen ion concentration.

IV.48 The intracellular fluid:

    A is approximately twice the volume of the extracellular fluid

    B the volume can be measured directly

    C is freely interchangeable with other body fluid compartments

    D contains approximately 150 mEq/L potassium

    E is a fairly constant fraction of all tissues

IV.49 Flow:

    A is the volume of fluid passing a point in unit time

    B in laminar flow, flow at the centre is about twice the mean rate and is approximately half the mean rate when in direct contact with the wall

    C under conditions of laminar flow, flow is directly proportional to pressure

    D halving the radius of the tube reduces flow to 1/16th of its original value

    E if the length of the tube is halved, flow will increase fourfold.

IV.50 Fluid and solute movement:

    A diffusion is proportional to the permeability of the membrane

    B an impermeable anion will hinder diffusion of a permeable cation

    C the Gibbs-Donnan equilibrium depends upon the presence of non-diffusible ions

    D the osmotic pressure is that necessary to prevent solute migration

    E filtration is hydrostatic pressure dependent.

IV.51 **Normal urinary electrolyte measurements include:**
  A   sodium 100 mmol/24 hours
  B   potassium 30 mmol/24 hours
  C   phosphate 30 mmol/24 hours
  D   calcium 5 mmol/24 hours
  E   urea 10 G/24 hours.

IV.52 **Gas chromatography:**
  A   depends on the partition of a substance between two
      phases, one stationary and one moving
  B   the stationary phase is an inert solid material that packs the
      column
  C   a specific detector is needed at the end of the column
  D   a particular gas can be identified by its specific profile
  E   the amount of a particular gas is calibrated against
      accurately known samples.

IV.53 **Electrical safety:**
  A   when touching faulty apparatus with wet hands, skin
      impedence is increased and current flow greater than
      normal
  B   electrical shock is not a risk with potentials below 24V AC or
      50V DC
  C   the modern diathermy earthing plate is not connected
      directly to earth
  D   microshock may lead to ventricular fibrillation via an
      intracardiac catheter with currents in excess of 150
      microamps
  E   leakage currents are induced voltages in other circuits
      resulting from an alternating mains current.

IV.54 **Suction apparatus:**
  A   the larger the reservoir, the higher the suction that is
      developed
  B   the smaller the reservoir, the more rapidly can suction be
      developed
  C   the maximal suction pressure developed should be about
      two-thirds of an atmosphere
  D   a long narrow suction catheter will reduce the flow but
      increase the applied suction pressure
  E   suction apparatus should achieve a free flow of 40 litres of
      air per minute.

IV.55 **Flow:**
  A   if Reynold's number exceeds 1000, turbulent flow is likely to
      be present
  B   the critical velocity at which laminar flow changes to
      turbulent flow varies only with the gas involved
  C   helium reduces the density of inspired gases and therefore
      the likelihood of turbulent flow within the respiratory tract
  D   turbulent flow within blood vessels is only detectable by
      invasive techniques
  E   endotracheal tube adaptors (e.g. Magill, Cobb) are
      specifically designed to avoid turbulent flow.

IV.56 Boyle's law:

A concerns a fixed mass of gas
B applies by definition to ideal gases only
C states that at constant temperature volume varies directly with pressure
D can be applied to vapours
E states that at constant volume pressure is directly proportional to absolute temperature.

IV.57 In pulmonary gas exchange:

A the PaO_2 is slightly lower than the PAO_2 because equilibration at each alveolus is not quite complete
B the $PACO_2$ is virtually independent of pulmonary blood flow in normal subjects
C the PAN_2 is 74 kPa
D the PAO_2 is directly proportional to atmospheric pressure
E the diffusion coefficient of oxygen is lower than that of carbon dioxide.

IV.58 Isotopes:

A are atoms with the same number of protons but different numbers of electrons
B are atoms with the same number of protons but different numbers of neutrons
C of the same element are chemically identical
D of the same element have different mass numbers
E cannot be separated physically.

IV.59 Temperature:

A the SI unit of temperature in the kelvin
B 1 kelvin is 1/273.16 of the thermodynamic temperature of the triple point of water
C mercury thermometers are suitable for temperatures down to −60°C
D alcohol thermometers tend to be non-linear
E the Bourdon gauge can be adapted to measure temperature.

IV.60 The following are true:

A temperature is not a form of energy
B using resistance wire temperature can be measured to 10^{-4}°C
C thermistors are accurate but have a slow response time
D thermocouples depend on the Seebeck effect
E the absolute calibration for temperature is the triple point of water.

Paper IV Answers

IV.1 TFTFT

- **B** Intracellular bicarbonate concentration is 10–20 mmol/L.
- **D** Approx 23 L, one third of the body weight in kilograms.
- **E** True, in potassium depletion intracellular H+ rises and bicarbonate is conserved to compensate

IV.2 FFTFT

- **A** An amino-acid, not an end-product.
- **B** From nucleotide bases, not proteins.
- **D** In man, ammonia is converted to urea, mainly in the liver.
- **E** From the sulphur-containing amino-acids: cysteine and methionine.

IV.3 FTFFF

- **C** No reaction is 100% efficient. Aerobic oxidation is 60% efficient, the rest produces heat.
- **D** From carbohydrate and protein metabolism, not fat.
- **E** RQ=CO_2 output / O_2 uptake. RQ for carbohydrates is higher (1.0 cf 0.7) for exactly the opposite reason: you can check this from a consideration of the molecular formulae of carbohydrates and fats.

IV.4 TTTTT

All these are the normal compensatory reactions to the fall in venous return and blood pressure and the hydrostatic changes that occur on standing.

IV.5 TFTTF

- **B** A bad question: does it mean at rest and in the change from a young to an old adult, or from childhood to adult? – probably the former, in which case the answer is probably false. Perhaps it would be better not to answer.
- **E** Increases in fever.

IV.6   TFFTF
   B   Chemical, not electrical transmission.
   C   Serotonin (5-HT) is a transmitter in the lateral grey horns of the spinal cord, the brain stem and hypothalamus
   E   Gamma efferent motor fibres.

IV.7   FTTTT
   A   85%

IV.8   TFFTF
   C   The cellular action is at ribosomal level. Some of the actions of growth hormone are mediated via somatomedins.
   E   Alpha-no; beta-yes.

IV.9   FFFFT
   A   The enkephalins are short-chain peptides: beta-endorphin contains 31 residues. Beta-endorphin is a component of beta-lipotropin that itself arises from a yet larger polypepetide precursor.
   B   Mu – brain; kappa – spinal cord; sigma – dysphoria. No doubt further research will produce new receptors and further sub-divisions of the receptors known already.
   C   Present throughout the CNS.
   D   Increased during exercise.

IV.10 TFTTT
   B   Sodium-potassium-activated ATPase.

IV.11 TTTFT

    D   Stimulated by steroids.

IV.12 TTTFF

    D   PTT >30secs.

    E   Euglobulin clot lysis time >30mins.

IV.13 FFFFF

In unmyelinated fibres, velocity is proportional to the square root of the diameter; in myelinated fibres, velocity is proportional directly to the diameter. Velocity is decreased by cold.

    A   Decreased by pressure. Pressure eventually causes failure of conduction.

    B,C Altering ionic concentrations in a preparation in vitro can certainly affect whether an impulse is propagated or not but the velocity of an impulse, once propagated, is affected very little. There is no effect in vivo.

    D   Not universally true: it depends on which motor and sensory nerves are being compared.

    E   Unaffected.

IV.14 TTFTF

    C   ADH acts on the distal convoluted tubule and collecting duct.

    E   The receptors are in the anterior hypothalamus and appear to be separate from the supra-optic and paraventricular nuclei.

IV.15 TFTTF

    B   Increased, leading to water retention and oedema.

    E   Increased.

IV.16 TFTTF

B   Dead space increases with tidal volume, mainly because the large airways expand.

C   "Ideal" alveolar gas is a concept only: arterial and mixed expired gas would have this same composition if there were no dead space or shunt.

E   Meaningless in this context: an example of "diffusion limitation" would be the transfer of carbon monoxide in the lung.

IV.17 TTTFF

D   Rubbish!

E   True, the membrane contains pores, but these are between alveoli to facilitate passage of gas from one to another.

IV.18 TTTFT

B   Because of cerebral vasoconstriction.

D   ICP is reduced, but via a fall in blood flow.

E   Hypocapnia causes alkalaemia, H^+ retention and consequent Na^- loss.

IV.19 TFTTT

A,D,E From a consideration of the oxyhaemoglobin dissociation curve.

B   Content does not affect saturation: an anaemic patient can have blood that is fully saturated. (Further knowledge will show that 2,3-DPG levels are increased in anaemia, but that is not the basic principle being tested here.)

IV.20 TTFTF

You should be able to draw a graph of the intra-thoracic pressures and volume over the respiratory cycle.

C   Intragastric will measure intra-abdominal pressure. A lower oesophageal balloon will reflect intra-pleural pressure.

D   It is higher (ie less negative) for simple, gravitational, reasons.

E   Forced expiration increases pressure above atmospheric. The alveoli can only be at atmospheric pressure if there is no air flow.

IV.21 FTFFF

A,D,E Inhibitors of protein synthesis within the cell at the level of the bacterial ribosome.

C Active metabolite, sulphanilamide, competes with para-amino benzoic acid, producing metabolic inhibition

IV.22 TTTFT

A Prolongs diastolic perfusion time.

C True, may produce hypoglycaemia.

D Slight reduction or unchanged.

IV.23 TTFFT

C No – increases both respiratory rate and tidal volume.

D No effect or possible mild bronchodilation.

IV.24 FTTTF

The best treatment is cardioversion. Otherwise, lignocaine is a reasonable first choice, with procainamide as an alternative. Disopyramide is also effective.

A Digoxin is contra-indicated.

E Verapamil ("Cordilox") is used in angina and supraventricular tachycardias. It slows AV conduction by inhibiting calcium transfer.

IV.25 TTTFT

B Initial hypertension following intravenous administration is probably caused by noradrenaline release from labile stores.

D May last for up to 7 days.

E True, although reduction in sympathetic activity may allow relative parasympathetic overactivity.

IV.26 TTFTT
- **B**   An anticholinesterase which crosses the blood-brain barrier.
- **C**   Does not cross the blood-brain barrier.
- **D**   A mild stimulant, large doses may convulse. Related to amphetamines. Sometimes used to try to abolish hiccough.
- **E**   Analeptic with a non-specific arousal effect.

IV.27 TTFTF
- **C**   Anti-diabetes insipidus effect – decreased free water clearance leads to decreased osmolality and perhaps decreased thirst.
- **E**   Hypokalaemia.

IV.28 FTFTT
- **A**   Intralipid is not irritant.
- **B**   Side-effects include nausea in 10%, headache, fever and palpitations.
- **E**   Each litre contains 200G of fat emulsion, plus 11G of glycerol to aid tonicity.

IV.29 FTFTF
- **A**   Chemically from malonic acid and urea, not uric acid.
- **B**   Up to a point: with the longer side chains and very high fat solubilities they become toxic and convulsant.
- **C**   In the 1930's.
- **E**   Look up the formulae.

IV.30 TTTTT
- **A**   Theoretically! We would not choose open ether if a relaxant method were available, and if caution dictated a gaseous induction then would choose halothane.
- **B**   It has an inhibitory action on descending pathways, as do all general anaesthetics, but also has an action at the neuromuscular junction.

IV.31 FTTFF

> A   It is an isomer of enflurane, but it is a fluorinated methyl-ethyl ether.
>
> C   Respiratory depression: halothane < isoflurane < enflurane.
>
> D   Blood:gas = 1.4. (Enflurane 1.91, halothane 2.5).
>
> E   Depression of BP is rather more than with halothane but the myocardial depression is less.

IV.32 TFFTF

> B   It will be different because venous blood is more acid, but not markedly so.
>
> D,E   It will slow secretion but not prevent it, but it will prevent "rapid" filtration.

IV.33 FTFFT

If the plasma concentration is high enough then any drug will cross the blood-brain barrier, but one must answer these questions sensibly.

> A   Aminoglycosides are highly polar and little accumulates in the CNS. Remember, though, that they are ototoxic.
>
> C   Not readily when the meninges are normal.
>
> D   Highly polar.

IV.34 FFTTF

> A   Cyclopropane is associated with bronchoconstriction.
>
> B   Trichloroethylene has no effect on the bronchi.
>
> E   Nitrous oxide has no effect on the bronchi.

IV.35 FTFTT

> A   Streptokinase activates plasminogen and stimulates fibrinolysis.
>
> C   Plasmin is activated to plasminogen, a proteinase.

IV.36 TFTTT

> Almost all local anaesthetics cause direct vasodilatation, although procaine is the only one in which it is clinically significant (it shortens its duration of action markedly).
>
> **B**   Cocaine causes local vasoconstiction because it potentiates the action of adrenaline by blocking re-uptake at sympathetic nerve terminals.

IV.37 FTTFT

> Either by being metabolised by pseudocholinesterase themselves **(B)** or being an inhibitor **(C,E)**. Lignocaine and atropine have no effect, though atropine is used to moderate the muscarinic actions of suxamethonium.

IV.38 FFTFT

> **A**   Many are totally synthetic.
> **B**   There are specific receptors: this is a very big, new, and advancing field.
> **D**   They are frequently poorly absorbed when taken orally, but that does not make them inactive.
> **E**   Butyrophenones are major tranquillizers.

IV.39 TTTFT

> **D**   No – it is incompatible in vitro.

IV.40 TFTTT

> **B**   Vagal stimulation leading to bradycardia: not, therefore, "confidently", but "with care".
> **C**   True, alpha-methyldopa does not produce elevated levels of either direct or indirect acting amines.
> **E**   True, cefuroxime is not an aminoglycoside.

IV.41 TTFFF

    C   It should be stored on ice until measured (and that as soon as possible).

    D   It should be withdrawn into an already heparinised syringe.

    E   The lowest strength heparin is sufficient: the higher strengths may alter the pH of the sample.

IV.42 TFTTT

    B   Too narrow a cuff produces artificially elevated measurements.

    D   Doppler frequency shift is caused by red cell movement.

IV.43 TFFTT

    B   Physiological IS the total dead space.

    C   No – this measures anatomical dead space.

    D,E   Both true. Bohr's equation states that: $PeCO_2 \times Vt = PaCO_2 \times (Vt-Vd) + PiCO_2 \times Vd$.

IV.44 TTFTT

    C   Used fairly specifically for halothane analysis in anaesthesia and are unaffected by nitrous oxide, carbon dioxide or water vapour

IV.45 TTFTF

    A   The low end of the normal range.

    C   This will sample dead space air!

    E   No, normal quiet respiration.

IV.46 FTFTT

A   A paired t-test is more powerful than an unpaired t-test, but paired tests *per se* are not necessarily more powerful tests.

C   The confidence limits of a mean can be calculated from the SEM in the same way that the confidence limits of a set of observations can be calculated from the mean and standard deviation.

IV.47 TTFTF

A   This follows from the law of Mass Action and the dissociation constant of water. Strictly the temperature should be defined as well **B**.

C   No: as PCO_2 increases, pH decreases.

D   The activity is less than the concentration in concentrated solutions.

E   1 pH unit = 10 fold.

IV.48 TFTTF

B   It can only be measured by knowing the total body water and subtracting the extracellular fluid volume.

E   This is true of lean body tissues but not of fat.

IV.49 TFTTF

B   Flow at the wall is zero.

E   Halving the length of the tube will double flow.

IV.50 TTTFT

D   SOLVENTmigration.

What about gas or granules, etc etc.

IV.51 TFFTF

A	True – 70–160 mmol/24hours.
B	False – 40–120 mmol/24hours.
C	False – 6–20 mmol/24hours.
D	True – 2.5–7.5 mmol/24hours.

IV.52 TFTFT

B	The stationary phase is an organic solvent adsorbed onto the packing material.
C	The particular detector will depend on the gas to be measured.
D	There are no specific profiles. One must know what gas one is looking for and compare prepared standards of that gas.

IV.53 FTTTT

A	Skin impedence is reduced leading to greater current flow.

IV.54 FTTFT

A	The maximal suction is determined by the pump, not by the reservoir.
D	It reduces the flow because the pressure applied is reduced by the resistance of the catheter.

IV.55 FFTFF

A	Reynold's number is 2000, not 1000.
B	Critical velocity is also dependent upon the characteristics of the tube.
D	Auscultation of bruits, etc.
E	These adaptors produce a lot of turbulence.

IV.56 TTFFF

B   By definition this is true.
C   It is an inverse relation.
D   Strictly no, but it can be applied approximately.
E   This is true, but follows from Charles' law, not Boyle's.

IV.57 FTTTT

A   Right direction, wrong reason: it is ventilation-perfusion imbalance that is the reason. Equilibration may not be complete in severe exercise.
B   In normal subjects, the P_ACO_2 is proportional to the alveolar ventilation and the $PaCO_2$ is equal to the P_ACO_2.
D   This is true if other variables are constant.
E   This is true but has little physiological significance.

IV.58 FTTTF

A   In an atom, the number of protons always equals the number of electrons.
D,E They can be separated physically because they have different masses. (ie Mass number. Atomic number = protons: mass number = protons + neutrons.)

IV.59 TTFTT

C   Mercury solidifies at $-39°C$.
E   The Bourdon gauge can be filled with mercury or volatile liquid and directly calibrated to read temperature.

IV.60 TTFTF

A   Temperature is the thermal state and is analogous to activity. Heat is a form of energy. The direction of net heat flow depends on the relative temperatures of two bodies not the total quantity of heat. (Consider a red hot pin dropped into a bucket of boiling water.)
C   Accurate, true, but thermistors have a fast response.
D   A temperature-sensitive voltage produced at the contact of two dissimilar metals.
E   The triple point is used to construct the Kelvin scale, but the absolute calibration of temperature is the hydrogen thermometer.

Paper V   Questions

V.1   **The vesicles in the adrenal medulla:**
   A   contain isoprenaline
   B   catecholamines are bound to chromogranin
   C   contain DOPA decarboxylase
   D   calcium ions are involved in the release process
   E   release is cholinergic and is blocked by atropine.

V.2   **The following are mitochondrial enzymes:**
   A   cytochrome oxidase
   B   lactate dehydrogenase
   C   chymotrypsin
   D   succinate dehydrogenase
   E   arginase.

V.3   **Concerning calcium:**
   A   serum concentration is increased by parathormone
   B   approximately half the serum calcium is non-diffusible
   C   the non-diffusible serum fraction is mostly as relatively insoluble salts
   D   the tendency to tetany is proportional to the ratio of calcium to magnesium ions
   E   tetany arises because of interference with neuromuscular transmission.

V.4   **Physiological right to left shunt (venous admixture) is:**
   A   partly flow from bronchial veins into pulmonary veins
   B   partly from Thebesian veins
   C   20% of total pulmonary blood flow
   D   increased by pulmonary hypertension
   E   increased during sleep.

V.5   **The function of the elastic tissue within the aortic wall is:**
   A   to prevent the aorta expanding with each beat
   B   to maintain the onward flow of blood during ventricular diastole
   C   to minimise the effects of intrathoracic pressure upon aortic pressure
   D   to convert intermittent to continuous blood flow with minimal pressure loss
   E   to maintain coronary perfusion.

V.6   The stretch reflex:

A   the knee-jerk is a monosynaptic reflex
B   the latency of the human knee jerk is 200 msec
C   stretch reflexes in the decerebrate cat, transected below the superior colliculi, are chiefly present in flexors
D   a stretch reflex is when muscle stretch activates a reflex arc which contracts the same muscle
E   a stretch reflex is when stretching a muscle causes a reflex increase of tone in that muscle.

V.7   Magnesium:

A   is the second most abundant intracellular cation
B   approximately half the total body content is in bone
C   is important in neuromuscular activity
D   growth hormone increases plasma magnesium
E   reduces peripheral vascular tone.

V.8   The following are true:

A   thyroxine is a substituted amino acid
B   prostaglandins are fatty acids
C   steroids have their cellular effects via protein synthesis
D   the peptide hormones are derived from beta-lipotrophin
E   corticosterone is the principal glucocorticoid in man.

V.9   Aldosterone secretion:

A   is reduced during surgery
B   is increased due to inferior vena caval compression
C   decreases on standing
D   is reduced in cases of low sodium intake
E   is only secreted in conjunction with glucocorticoid release.

V.10   Cell membranes:

A   are normally composed of a single lipid layer between two layers of protein
B   lipid soluble substances cross membranes in proportion to their lipid-water partition coefficient
C   water soluble substances penetrate membranes in proportion to molecular size
D   ionisation decreases fat solubility
E   degree of ionisation is solely dependent upon the pK of the substance.

V.11 Mechanisms necessary for normal haemostasis include:
- A activation of the kallikrein-kinin system
- B blood flow diversion due to altered local haemodynamics
- C fibrinolysis
- D the acute phase response
- E factor XIII.

V.12 Adverse drug reactions may be due to:
- A idiosyncrasy
- B hypersensitivity
- C angioneurotic oedema
- D serum sickness
- E secondary effects.

V.13 Nerve fibres:
- A have a lower electrical resistance than surrounding body fluids and tissues
- B the velocity of propagation of the impulse is faster in larger fibres
- C the fastest conduction velocities are about 100 metres per second
- D pain fibres are unmyelinated and are A-delta and C fibres
- E smaller fibres are less susceptible to local anaesthetics.

V.14 Concerning body sodium:
- A the major losses are by sweating
- B the kidney will have adjusted to a change in intake within 16 hours
- C reabsorption of sodium is mainly in the DCT where it is stimulated by aldosterone
- D about 22,000 mEq of sodium are filtered each day
- E in hyperaldosteronism there is always a positive sodium balance.

V.15 Tubular reabsorption:
- A 7/8ths of all reabsorption occurs within the proximal tubule
- B sodium reabsorption is mainly passive
- C the sodium pump is inhibited by ethacrynic acid
- D active proximal tubular reabsorption may be transport – maximum limited
- E if the tubular walls are permeable to the solute, active reabsorption will be gradient-time limited.

V.16   Carbon dioxide:

A   causes dilation of cerebral blood vessels

B   the normal content of arterial blood is about 48 volumes per cent

C   affects the excitability of neurones in the reticular activating system

D   has a tension in mixed venous blood 0.8 kPa (6 mm Hg) higher than in arterial blood

E   aids displacement of oxygen from haemoglobin.

V.17   The PIO2:

A   is approximately 19.9 kPa (149 mm Hg) in air saturated with water vapour at 37°C

B   can be increased by hyperventilation

C   is linearly related to the concentration of oxygen in the inspired air

D   is one of the terms in the alveolar air equation

E   is used to calculate ventilatory dead space.

V.18   Which of the following statements are true:

A   the carotid and aortic bodies are sensitive to arterial blood pressure

B   hypotension produces increased baroreceptor discharge

C   increased plasma renin activity stimulates aldosterone production

D   posture influences aldosterone production

E   antidiuretic hormone secretion is influenced by baroreceptor activity.

V.19   Adult human haemoglobin:

A   is a tetramer

B   the molecule changes shape during oxygenation

C   98% is HbA

D   HbF may be present in otherwise normal individuals

E   has a molecular weight of about 65,000.

V.20   Pulmonary surfactant:

A   increases surface tension differentially in different sized alveoli

B   helps prevent pulmonary oedema

C   increases alveolar ciliary motion

D   aids diffusion from the alveolus to the pulmonary capillary

E   is produced by the type II alveolar cells.

V.21   The following do not adversely affect the foetus:

    A streptomycin

    B cloxacillin

    C tetracycline

    D tobramycin

    E cefuroxime.

V.22   The following drugs can cause an increase in blood pressure:

    A phentolamine

    B guanethidine

    C thymoxamine

    D propranolol

    E bethanidine.

V.23   **Ephedrine:**

    A is both a direct and indirect acting sympathomimetic amine

    B has both alpha and beta effects

    C is a monoamine-oxidase inhibitor

    D may induce bronchoconstriction

    E reduces renal blood flow due to local vasoconstriction.

V.24   The following are positive inotropic agents:

    A labetolol

    B isoprenaline

    C protamine

    D prilocaine

    E calcium ions.

V.25   **Dobutamine:**

    A has structural characteristics of both dopamine and
        isoprenaline

    B is a synthetic sympathomimetic amine

    C is a selective beta–1 stimulant

    D produces an increase in cardiac output without significant
        chronotropic effect

    E stimulates dopaminergic receptors in the kidney.

V.26   The following induce epileptiform EEG activity:

    A   enflurane
    B   midazolam
    C   methohexitone
    D   etomidate
    E   isoflurane.

V.27   Metabolic acidosis inhibits the diuretic action of:

    A   triamterene
    B   mersalyl
    C   frusemide
    D   chlorothiazide
    E   acetazolamide.

V.28   Sodium nitroprusside:

    A   the maximum safe intraoperative dose rate should not
         exceed 10 micrograms/kg/min
    B   metabolism to cyanide occurs non-enzymatically in blood
    C   metabolism produces thiocyanate which is excreted in urine
    D   produces dilation of both resistance and capacitance vessels
    E   administration is contraindicated in tobacco amblyopia.

V.29   Thiopentone:

    A   is formulated as the sodium salt to make it soluble in water
    B   in solution, as available, has a high pH
    C   acts in one arm-brain circulation time
    D   can be injected intra-arterially with care
    E   has a pK approximately the same as the normal pH of
         plasma.

V.30   Methoxyflurane:

    A   is an analgesic in sub-anaesthetic concentrations
    B   has a MAC in man of 0.45%
    C   is more soluble in blood than is halothane
    D   is potentially nephrotoxic
    E   may interact with diuretics.

V.31 Nitrous oxide:

A forms a reversible complex with haemoglobin
B may induce teratogenicity following prolonged exposure in pregnant rats
C induces diffusion hypoxia
D may induce postoperative deafness
E interferes with vitamin B_{12} metabolism in the liver.

V.32 The absorption of weak acids from the stomach:

A is at a rate directly proportional to the pH of gastric juice
B is faster than that of weak bases
C the unionised acid diffuses across the gastric mucosa
D is reduced in achlorhydria
E occurs during secretion of gastric acid induced by gastrin but not histamine.

V.33 Centrally acting anti-emetics include:

A metoclopramide
B perphenazine
C hyoscine
D cyclizine
E droperidol.

V.34 Anticonvulsant activity is associated with:

A clonazepam
B chlormethiazole
C thiopentone
D ketamine
E chlorpromazine.

V.35 Contraction of the pregnant uterus is stimulated by:

A progesterone
B vasopressin
C ergotamine
D histamine
E salbutamol.

V.36   Amethocaine: Tetracaine.

- **A** is hydrolysed by plasma cholinesterase
- **B** has a quinidine-like effect on the heart
- **C** maximum dose should not exceed 3 mg/kg
- **D** a standard amethocaine lozenge contains 65 mg
- **E** is rapidly inactivated in acidic surroundings.

V.37   Dantrolene:

- **A** relaxes muscle by making calcium readily available at the cellular level
- **B** given orally may protect a susceptible individual
- **C** intravenous dosage is 300 mg/kg
- **D** causes muscle weakness
- **E** depresses polysynaptic reflexes.

V.38   Which of these statements are true:

- **A** paracetamol causes gastric erosions
- **B** indomethacin is a conjugated salicylate
- **C** aspirin lowers normal body temperature
- **D** phenylbutazone can precipitate cardiac failure
- **E** mefanamic acid causes diarrhoea.

V.39   Morphine:

- **A** is a phenanthrene derivative
- **B** may produce increased parasympathetic tone
- **C** has an anticholinergic effect
- **D** decreases cerebrospinal fluid pressure
- **E** is a good anticonvulsant.

V.40   The following drugs should be avoided in patients with severe renal impairment (GFR<10 ml/min):

- **A** digoxin
- **B** metformin
- **C** gallamine
- **D** disopyramide
- **E** sulphadiazine.

V.41 The weight of gas dissolved in a liquid at constant ambient pressure at equilibrium depends on:
- **A** temperature of the liquid
- **B** partial pressure of the gas
- **C** diffusion coefficient
- **D** solubility of the gas in the liquid
- **E** critical temperature of the gas.

V.42 Direct blood pressure measurement:
- **A** the lowest frequency normally measured is related to heart rate, the lower limit being 0.5 Hz
- **B** the upper frequency limit of suitable measuring apparatus should be 10 Hz
- **C** the peak systolic pressure in the dorsalis pedis artery is 10% higher than that in the aorta
- **D** the resonant frequency of the system may be raised by using a shorter and stiffer catheter
- **E** critical damping must be used if the system is to be accurate.

V.43 The normal partial pressure of:
- **A** oxygen in the alveoli is 100 mm Hg (13.3 kPa)
- **B** nitrogen in inspired air is 596 mm Hg (79.5 kPa)
- **C** water vapour in the alveoli is 40 mm Hg (5.3 kPa)
- **D** carbon dioxide in mixed expired gas is 32 mm Hg (4.3 kPa)
- **E** oxygen in the right heart is 40 mm Hg (5.3 kPa).

V.44 A refractometer:
- **A** is capable of measuring vapour concentrations in known gas mixtures
- **B** does not require prior calibration
- **C** can provide a direct measurement of percentage concentration
- **D** is uninfluenced by water vapour in the gas mixture
- **E** is a commonly used calibration method in the manufacture of vaporisers.

V.45 Linear regression analysis:
- **A** applies a technique of minimising squared differences
- **B** can apply to variables that are not distributed normally
- **C** yields a regression coefficient (the gradient)
- **D** the intercepts will define the position of the line
- **E** the correlation coefficent is an indication of the "goodness of fit" of the line to the data.

V.46 Errors in statistics:

 A   a Type I error is when the test predicts wrongly that an
      observation is from a different population
 B   a Type I error is the acceptance that some values that lie
      outside p<0.05 may well be from that distribution
 C   a Type II error is when the test predicts wrongly that an
      observation is from the same population
 D   a Type II error is the probability (beta) of not finding a
      positive result when one actually exists
 E   Type I and Type II errors can be reduced by making trials
      double-blind.

V.47 The carriage of CO_2 by the blood:

 A   is 85% as bicarbonate
 B   is partly as carboxyhaemoglobin
 C   influences the affinity of haemoglobin for oxygen
 D   is approximately 48 vols per cent in arterial blood
 E   is aided in exercise by selective ionisation of amphoteric
      proteins.

V.48 The clearance of a solute:

 A   is the volume of plasma actually cleared of the solute
 B   is measured in ml/min
 C   is equal to the glomerular filtration rate
 D   is greater if the solute is secreted by the tubules
 E   is greater if the solute is osmotically active.

V.49 Colligative properties include or explain:

 A   the behaviour of azeotropes
 B   the depression of freezing point of a solvent by a solute
 C   the miscibility of different liquids
 D   the Choanda effect
 E   the effect of centrifugation on cell fractionation.

V.50 In cardioversion:

 A   it is the voltage that is important
 B   only 10–30% of the energy applied to the chest wall will pass
      through the myocardium
 C   direct current capacitor discharge is the preferred technique
 D   if alternating current is used it must be synchronised with
      the R wave
 E   the maximum energy applied should not exceed 100J.

V.51 Electrical safety:

A   operating theatre equipment is semi-conductive to allow static electricity to drain away

B   operating theatre floors have a very low resistance to prevent static charge building up

C   antistatic charge is conducted through carbon based materials

D   endotracheal tubes are rendered conductive by the high humidity of gases passing through them

E   cotton possesses antistatic properties.

V.52 The following are true statements about flow:

A   at constant pressure, flow is directly proportional to resistance

B   laminar flow is inversely proportional to viscosity

C   doubling the radius of a tube lowers the resistance to flow by l/16th

D   in turbulent flow the velocity is greatest at the periphery of the column of fluid

E   resistance to flow in a tube varies directly as the length.

V.53 Concerning the Venturi principle:

A   flowing gas contains energy as potential energy which is manifested as pressure

B   flowing gas contains kinetic energy which is manifested as flow rate

C   in a venturi, at the point of narrowing, flow increases and potential energy increases

D   in a venturi, at the point of constriction, pressure falls

E   beyond the venturi constriction, kinetic energy falls and potential energy and pressure rise.

V.54 If a liquid is allowed to vaporise in a mixture of gases to equilibrium, the partial pressure of the vapour in the mixture will depend on:

A   the volume of the liquid

B   the temperature of the liquid

C   the surface area of the liquid

D   atmospheric pressure

E   the liquid density.

V.55 Nitrous oxide:

A   is produced commercially by heating ammonium nitrate to 240° C

B   gas is stored in metal cylinders at 51 atmospheres

C   nitric oxide and nitrogen dioxide may be present in small amounts

D   is 15 times more soluble than oxygen in blood

E   blood/gas partition coefficient is 0.47.

V.56 In the estimate of the arterial PCO$_2$:

A the Fick principle can be used

B the end-tidal PCO$_2$ is a good estimate in fit healthy subjects

C the end-tidal PCO$_2$ is not a good estimate in infants because of the higher metabolic rate

D the rebreathing technique relies on equilibration between arterial and mixed venous PCO$_2$

E Astrup interpolation depends on constructing buffer lines.

V.57 Explosions:

A mixtures are ignited 100 times more easily in oxygen than in air

B diethyl ether will burn in 1.5% nitrous oxide in air

C the "zone of risk" is within 25 cm of the patient

D antistatic rubber anaesthetic tubing should have a resistance of at least 25 K Ohms per 5 ft

E to avoid explosions, the relative humidity in theatres should be maintained at 35%.

V.58 Temperature:

A the electrical resistance of metal increases linearly with temperature

B the resistance of metal oxides used in thermistors falls as temperature rises

C the resistance change in a thermistor is exponentially related to temperature

D a thermocouple depends upon voltage change occurring in response to the temperature at the junction of two dissimilar metals

E unlike other devices, thermistors can routinely be heat sterilised.

V.59 Humidity and humidifiers:

A the ideal humidity to avoid risk of explosion is 100%

B absolute humidity is constant at a given temperature and pressure

C can be measured using a Regnault's hygrometer

D nebulised droplets should ideally be 20 microns in diameter

E it is impossible to attain a relative humidity of more than 100%.

V.60 Regarding computers:

A a digital computer can only accept numerical input

B a bit is a binary digit

C ensure mathematical accuracy

D a program is a series of instructions

E an analogue computer could be used to construct an electrical model of a physiological process.

Paper V Answers

V.1 FTFTF

A   Isoprenaline is a synthetic catecholamine.

C   This enzyme converts DOPA (dihydroxyphenylalanine) to dopamine, which then enters the granules.

E   Release is cholinergic, but is not blocked by atropine.

V.2 TFFTF

A   Respiratory chain oxidation.

B   A cytoplasmic enzyme that exists in 5 forms or isoenzymes and catalyses the interconversion of pyruvate and lactate.

C   In exocrine pancreatic secretions.

D   In the citric acid cycle.

E   In the urea cycle: catalyses the irreversible hydrolysis of arginine to yield urea and regenerate ornithine.

V.3 TTFFF

C   The non-diffusible fraction is protein-bound rather than ionised: 75% to albumin, 25% to globulin.

D   The tendency to tetany = $([HCO_3^-][HPO_4^{2-}])/([Ca^{2+}][Mg^{2+}][H^+])$.

E   Tetany is caused by an increase in motor nerve activity that overrides

DEPRESSION of transmission at the neuromuscular junction.

V.4 TTFFT

B   Thebesian veins drain directly into the heart chambers.

C   About 2%.

D   Shunt may well be increased in the conditions that give rise to pulmonary hypertension, but pulmonary hypertension does not, per se, increase venous admixture.

V.5 FTFFT

A   The aorta stretches during systole.

C   Maybe a bit but not the intended answer.

D   Intermittent flow persists far further down the arterial tree.

V.6   TFTTF
B   20–25 msec.
C   True, local stimulation will cause flexion of the ipsilateral and extension of the contralateral side.
E   Tone control is mediated through gamma efferents.

V.7   TTTFF
D   Lowers serum magnesium by stimulating retention in bone and soft tissues.
E   True; magnesium produces peripheral vasodilation and hypotension.

V.8   TTTFF
A   Thyroxine is tetraiodothyronine.
D   SOME may be, but not all.
E   Cortisol is the principle glucocorticoid, approximately 7 times as much is secreted in 24 hours, and plasma concentration is approximately 30 times higher than, corticosterone.

V.9   FTFFF
A   Mildly increased.
C   Increases secondary to renin secretion in response to hypotension.
D   Elevated to retain sodium.
E   Secreted alone in situations of electrolyte imbalance.

V.10   FTTTF
A   Bilipid layer sandwiched between protein.
E   Local pH and pK together.

V.11 TTTTF

    E   Fibrin stabilising factor – not necessary in the initial stages of haemostasis

V.12 TTFFT

    C,D   Both these are symptoms, not causes.

V.13 FTTFF

    A   The simple electrical resistance of the membrane, like all membranes, is very high. It is the controlled changes in membrane permeabilities that enable nervous transmission.

    B   In unmyelinated fibres, velocity is proportional to the square root of the diameter; in myelinated fibres, velocity is proportional directly to the diameter.

    D   True of pain fibres – but A-delta fibres are myelinated.

    E   Smaller fibres are more susceptible to local anaesthetics.

V.14 FFFTF

    A   The major losses under normal circumstances are in the urine.

    B   3 days: the implication is total adjustment, not partial.

    C   It is true that reabsorption is stimulated by aldosterone in the DCT but 90% of the reabsorption is in the PCT and loop of Henle.

    E   A new steady-state will be reached in which total body sodium is abnormally high.

V.15 TFTTT

    B   Mainly active in proximal tubule.

V.16 TTTTT

    B CO_2 is much more soluble than oxygen: blood contains more and at a lower partial pressure.

    C   Initially excitation, eventually CO_2 narcosis.

    D   This figure is used in the rebreathing method of estimating $PaCO_2$.

V.17 TFTTF

    A   (Ambient pressure – SVP of water) $\times$ FiO_2.

    B   The ALVEOLAR oxygen tension, but not the inspired oxygen tension, can be increased by hyperventilation.

    C   The law of partial pressures.

    D $PaO_2 = PiO_2 - PaCO_2/R - F$. R=respiratory quotient, F=nitrogen correction.

    E   The Bohr equation uses carbon dioxide not oxygen.

V.18 FFTTT

    A   Carotid and aortic bodies contain chemoreceptors, the baroreceptors are situated in carotid sinus and aortic arch.

    B   Hypertension increases baroreceptor discharge, which in turn inhibits tonic discharge of vasoconstrictor nerves and excites the cardio-inhibitory centre.

V.19 TTTTT

    A   A tetramer is a molecule with 4 sub-units. Myoglobin is a monomer.

    B   The beta chains move relative to one another.

    C   2% is HbA2.

V.20 FTFFT

    A   It DECREASES surface tension inversely with lung volume

    B   The high surface tension would otherwise be a force drawing water in.

    D   It has no effect, per se, on diffusion.

V.21 FTFFT

- **A** Ototoxic.
- **C** Deposited in bones and teeth.
- **D** Aminoglycosides are generally contraindicated in pregnancy because of the risk of renal and eighth nerve damage.

V.22 FTFFT

- **A** Alpha adrenergic blocker.
- **B** Vasodilator. Although primarily hypotensive, initial intravenous administration causes HYPERtension due to release of transmitter from labile stores.
- **C** Alpha adrenergic blocker.
- **D** Beta blocker – hypertension may occur but only on withdrawal of drug.

V.23 TTTFT

- **D** Bronchodilation due to inhibition of bronchial muscle.
- **E** True, kidney blood flow is not spared.

V.24 FTFFT

- **A** Labetolol (alpha and beta blocker) is a negative inotrope.
- **B** Isoprenaline is an almost pure beta agonist.
- **C** Protamine may cause bradycardia and hypotension, perhaps because of histamine release.
- **D** Most local anaesthetics depress the myocardium directly.

V.25 TTTTF

- **C,D** True, dobutamine is almost a pure inotrope.
- **E** Unlike dopamine, renal blood flow is not affected.

V.26   TFTFF
  B   Midazolam, being a benzodiazepine, is a CNS sedative.
  D   Etomidate is used as an anticonvulsant.
  E   Unlike enflurane, isoflurane has not been associated with
          convulsions.

V.27   FFFTT
  A   No – aldosterone antagonist.
  B   No – inhibited by metabolic alkalosis (see question 111.27)
  C   No – loop diuretic.

V.28   TTTTT
  E   Abnormality of cyanide metabolism.

V.29   TTTFT
  A   6 parts Na_2CO_3 to 100 parts thiopentone.
  D   If injected intra-arterially it causes intense pain and spasm
          in the arterioles severe enough to cause death of the
          tissues supplied.

V.30   TFTTF
  B   0.16%
  C   It is the most soluble agent currently available.
  D   Because of the release of free fluoride ions. It is dose-time
          related.

V.31 FTTTT

    A   Doesn't combine with haemoglobin.

V.32 FTTTF

The higher the pH, the more ionised will be the weak acid: absorption will thus be less. Consideration of this will explain options **A,D,C**, and **D**.

    E   Gastric acid is gastric acid no matter how its production is stimulated.

V.33 TTTTT

    D   True, cyclizine is a competitive antihistamine whose main action is on the vomiting centre.

V.34 TTTFF

    D,E   Careful, although neither possess CONVULSANT properties per se, they are not specifically used as anticonvulsants.

V.35 FTTTF

    A   Progesterone opposes the effect of oxytocin.

    C   Careful, the drug in clinical use is ergometrine, but ergotamine does have an effect too, though weaker.

    E   Is used to prevent premature labour.

V.36   TTFTF
Amethocaine:
C   The toxic and maximum dose is 100 mg per 70 kg.
E   Inactivated by alkalis.

V.37   FTFTF
A   Exactly the opposite: dantrolene uncouples
       excitation-contraction coupling.
C   1 mg/kg, repeated as necessary.
D   Yes: it may mean that IPPV is needed post-operatively.

V.38   FFFTT
B   An indole derivative, not a salicylate at all.
D   By fluid retention.
E   Mefenamic acid ("Ponstan") is as powerful an analgesic as
       aspirin but not as powerful an anti-inflammatory drug.

V.39   TTTFF
D   Increases, probably both directly and indirectly because of
       hypoventilation and carbon dioxide retention.
E   Morphine may produce excitation in some patients.

V.40   FTTFT
All these drugs should be used with caution in patients with
renal impairment but the question asks which should be
AVOIDED and quantifies the degree of impairment. According to
the British National Formulary:
A   Digoxin: up to 250 micrograms daily.
B   Metformin: avoid, risk of lactic acidosis.
C   Gallamine: avoid, prolonged blockade.
D   Disopyramide: reduce the dose.
E   Sulphadiazine: avoid, high risk of crystalluria.

V.41 TTFTF

- **A**   The higher the temperature, the lower the solubility.
- **B**   Henry's law.
- **C**   Irrelevant.
- **D**   Defined by either the Bunsen or the Ostwald solubility coefficient: the latter is the one more used in anaesthetic practice and is independent of the ambient pressure.
- **E**   Irrelevant.

V.42 TFTTF

- **B**   The upper frequency limit should be 30 Hz, related to the shape of the wave and the dicrotic notch.
- **E**   Critical damping is too severe for clinical use, the ideal is 70% of critical.

V.43 TTTTT

- **D**   Mixed expired gas is one that is often forgotten – P_EO_2 116(15.5), P_ECO_2 32(4.3), P_EH_2O 47(6.3) and P_EN_2 565(75) mm Hg (kPa)

V.44 TFTFT

- **B**   Does require prior calibration, particularly if a direct percentage concentration reading is required.
- **D**   Is affected by water vapour and is no good in circuits where water vapour concentration is changing.

V.45 TTTTT

- **B**   Strictly, the variables should be normally distributed. In practice, one can apply the analysis to some non-normal data.
- **E**   The correlation coefficient is usually denoted by a lower-case "r".

V.46 TTTTF

A,B Different expressions of the same idea.

C,D Different expressions of the same idea.

E This makes no difference: things like sample size and the expected variability of the observations affect the likelihood of these errors.

V.47 TFTTF

A CO_2 forms carbamino compounds with haemoglobin.

E This sounds very scientific and plausible but is nonsense. An amphoteric compound is one that can ionise to either donate or accept a hydrogen ion. Proteins are amphoteric because they have both carboxyl and amino groups that can ionise and this is one reason why they are effective buffers.

V.48 · FTTTF

A Clearance is a theoretical value and is the volume of plasma that contains the same quantity of the solute as is present in the volume of urine that is formed in one minute.

C Only if not secreted or absorbed by the tubules.

E A red herring: osmotic properties per se have no bearing on clearance or excretion.

V.49 TTFFF

Colligative properties are all related to osmolarity and include depression of freezing point, lowering of vapour pressure and raising of boiling point.

D The Choanda effect is the boundary-layer effect used in the operation of devices relying on fluidic logic.

V.50 FTTFF

A No, the current.

D AC cannot be synchronised, the discharge is too long (0.1–0.2 sec).

E Maximum recommended is 300J for an adult (though machines will usually discharge up to 400J), 150J for a child. Internal maximum is 80J for an adult.

V.51 TFFTT

  B   No, they must have sufficient resistance to prevent the
        passage of current and danger of electrocution.
  C   Careful – should be static, not antistatic, charge.

V.52 FTTFT

  A   This MUST be incorrect because, whatever the type of
        flow and the exact relation of flow to resistance, flow must
        DECREASE as resistance increases.
  B,C,E Follow from the Hagen-Poiseuille formula. If a question of
        this type occurs, write down the appropriate formula
        BEFORE the exact wording of the question can confuse
        you.
  D   Flow is always faster in the centre.

V.53 TTFTT

  C,D   Potential energy decreases and kinetic energy increases.

V.54 FTFFF

This is a re-statement of the meaning of saturated vapour
pressure: the nature of the liquid and the temperature only. If
only a small volume of liquid is introduced, then you could
argue that it would totally vaporise and not reach its SVP, in
other words that **A** is true. This is not so: the question is of a
state "in equilibrium" and implies that some of the liquid
remains as liquid.

V.55 TTFTT

  C   Certainly not routinely! A fatality occurred due to this in
        1966 (Clutton-Brock). The rest are facts that must be
        learned!

V.56 FTFFT

A CO_2 can be used as an indicator for measuring blood flow by the Fick principle, but Fick is not used to estimate $PaCO_2$.

C   The higher metabolic rate and higher respiratory frequency will cause a less well defined end-tidal plateau but the response time of the electrodes is fast enough to cope with this.

D   The equilibrium is between the bag and mixed venous blood. $PaCO_2$ is calculated on an assumption about the A-V CO_2 difference (6 mm Hg).

V.57 TTFTF

C   Within 25 cm of any part of the CIRCUIT.

D   This is the recommended figure for new tubing. Resistance rises with use and the recommendations are modified accordingly.

E   The higher the humidity the less the likelihood of sparks caused by static discharge, but high humidity is less comfortable to work in: a compromise figure of at least 50% is recommended.

V.58 TTTTF

E   Heat sterilisation alters the calibration.

V.59 TFTFF

A   This would, however, be very uncomfortable.

B   No! It depends on the mass of water vapour present and that is obviously variable.

D   20 microns: deposited in the trachea or URT, a nuisance
5 microns: deposited in the trachea
1 micron : deposited in the alveoli
<1 micron : ideal – not deposited, move in and out with airflow.

E   Supersaturation: a clinical risk of very efficient humidification.

V.60 FTFTT

A,B   A digital computer can handle many kinds of input. It is so named because the representation within the computer can only be as a series of bits that are either zero or 1

C,D   The computer will do, accurately, what it is told, but mathematical accuracy depends on the program being correct and that depends on the programmer – a human being!

Paper VI Questions

VI.1 The following are transmitters at autonomic ganglia:
  A dopamine
  B metacholine
  C GABA
  D 5-HT
  E glycine.

VI.2 Lactate dehydrogenase:
  A pyruvate is a substrate
  B catalyses the hydrolysis of lactose
  C is synthesised in skeletal muscle
  D requires ATP as coenzyme
  E is otherwise known as lactase.

VI.3 Calcium:
  A active uptake is enhanced by vitamin D
  B uptake is mainly in the terminal ileum
  C glucocorticoids raise plasma Ca^{2+} to cause osteoporosis
  D is present in bone mainly as hydroxyapatite
  E serum levels are lowered by calcitonin.

VI.4 The myocardium:
  A the cells have an internal resting potential of $+90$ mV
  B the intracellular potassium is about 150 mEq/L
  C the muscle cells form a syncitium
  D repolarises by the expulsion of sodium ions
  E does not metabolise lactate.

VI.5 Critical closing pressure is:
  A the elastic forces tending to close arteries
  B the elastic force tending to close veins
  C the pressure within a blood vessel at which it collapses down completely and is closed to flow
  D the activity of the precapillary sphincters
  E the external pressure required to prevent blood flow.

VI.6   The tendon jerks:

A   disappear if any part of their reflex arc is put out of action
B   are absent in cerebellar disease
C   are brisker in long motor tract damage
D   are increased on the ipsilateral side below the lesion in hemi
      section of the spinal cord
E   are inhibited by Ia afferents from Golgi tendon organs.

VI.7   Both bradykinin and histamine:

A   are direct vasodilators
B   increase capillary permeability
C   stimulate the secretion of gastric acid
D   cause pain when applied to a blister base
E   cause vasodilation in the axon reflex.

VI.8   Growth hormone:

A   is diabetogenic
B   its plasma half-life is 25 minutes
C   decreases fatty acid utilisation
D   shows only slight inter-species specificity
E   exerts all its effects via somatomedins.

VI.9   The following cause postoperative oliguria:

A   inappropriate ADH secretion
B   aldosterone
C   inadequate expansion of functional extracellular fluid
      volume
D   cortisol
E   high plasma renin activity.

VI.10   Gastric acid:

A   is isotonic
B   secretion is stimulated by anger, hypoglycaemia or gastric
      distension
C   is secreted by the parietal cells
D   secretion is abolished by vagotomy
E   gastrin and secretin form a regulatory feedback loop.

VI.11 The role of platelets in coagulation includes:
  A   adherence to exposed collagen
  B   vasoactive amine release
  C   inhibition of formation of thromboxane A2
  D   formation of prostaglandin endoperoxidase
  E   cycloxygenase inhibition.

VI.12 Antibody types:
  A   IgG is particularly extravascular
  B   IgM is the agglutinator antibody
  C   IgA is present in seromucous secretions
  D   high levels of reaginic antibody are always present in atopic
       individuals
  E   the antibody responsible for thiopentone hypersensitivity is
       likely to be an IgE type.

VI.13 These pathways correspond to the modalities:
  A   proprioception via the dorsal columns
  B   temperature and pain via the contralateral spinothalamic
       tracts
  C   fibres subserving fine touch cross then form the gracile and
       cuneate nuclei
  D   there is no overlap between adjacent segments
  E   referred pain is conducted via autonomic-somatic
       collaterals.

VI.14 The renal blood flow:
  A   is subject to autoregulation occuring mainly at the afferent
       arterioles
  B   is about one fifth of the cardiac output
  C   is independent of the renal nerves
  D   supplies a highly active organ that has a high unit oxygen
       extraction
  E   the glomerular filtration rate is independent of renal vascular
       resistance.

VI.15 Water excretion:
  A   180 litres of water are filtered daily
  B   if the obligatory solute load is excreted in 55 ml urine,
       osmolarity will be 1400 mosmol/L
  C   normal urine production is approximately 1 ml/kg/hour
  D   60% of water reabsorption occurs within the proximal tubule
  E   5% of water reabsorption occurs within the loop of Henle.

VI.16 At reduced body temperature:

A   oxygen and carbon dioxide are more soluble in body fluids
B   the oxyhaemoglobin dissociation curve shifts to the left
C   carbon dioxide carrying capacity is increased
D   oxygen requirements at 30°C are 70% of normal
E   blood viscosity is decreased.

VI.17 With increasing altitude:

A   the concentration of oxygen in the atmosphere falls
B   the atmospheric pressure decreases exponentially
C   water will boil at a temperature lower than 100°C
D $PaCO_2$ will decrease at first
E   acetazolamide can reduce the incidence of pulmonary oedema.

VI.18 Physiological dead space:

A   increases following induction of anaesthesia
B   decreases during controlled ventilation
C   increases with a short inspiration time
D   increases with the use of PEEP
E   is a dynamic lung volume.

VI.19 The oxyhaemoglobin dissociation curve is shifted to the right:

A   if foetal Hb is replaced by adult Hb
B   by an increase in 2,3-DPG in the erythrocytes
C   by a rise in temperature
D   by a rise in pH
E   by passage of blood through the lungs.

VI.20 When considering compliance of the lungs:

A   dynamic compliance can only be measured during IPPV
B   compliance is minimal during tidal breathing
C   compliance is increased at high lung volume
D   dynamic compliance can be said to be the same as chest wall compliance in a fit young adult
E   is 20 ml/cm H_2O in a normal individual.

VI.21 In man atropine causes:
- **A** secretion of anti-diuretic hormone
- **B** bradycardia
- **C** relaxation of uterine muscle
- **D** relaxation of ureteric muscle
- **E** mydriasis.

VI.22 Alpha adrenergic stimulation is the primary mode of action of:
- **A** phenylephrine
- **B** dopamine
- **C** methoxamine
- **D** isoprenaline
- **E** ephedrine.

VI.23 Metaraminol:
- **A** is a direct acting sympathomimetic amine
- **B** increases coronary blood flow
- **C** is a pure alpha agonist
- **D** produces a bradycardia
- **E** should not be given in conjunction with ganglion blocking drugs.

VI.24 Clonidine:
- **A** is used to treat migraine
- **B** reduces blood pressure by a direct venodilatation
- **C** is available in oral and parenteral preparations
- **D** sudden withdrawal may cause rebound hypertension
- **E** oral dosage is 3 to 36 mg daily.

VI.25 Warfarin:
- **A** competes with vitamin K
- **B** displaces phenylbutazone from plasma protein binding sites
- **C** blocks prothrombin synthesis
- **D** is contraindicated in malignant hypertension
- **E** prevents normal fibrinolysis.

VI.26 Intracranial pressure is increased by:
A halothane
B suxamethonium
C phenoperidine
D nitroglycerine
E etomidate.

VI.27 Hypochloraemic alkalosis:
A is best treated with ammonium hydroxide
B may be produced by mercurial diuretics
C is associated with a relative bicarbonate retention
D is produced by acetozolamide
E is associated with excessive urinary hydrogen ion excretion.

VI.28 Monoamine oxidase inhibitors include:
A tranylcypromine
B phenelzine
C dothiepin
D iproniazid
E fluphenazine.

VI.29 Methohexitone:
A is an oxy-barbiturate
B may cause pain on injection
C is methylated hexobarbitone
D is said to be safer than thiopentone in an asthmatic
E is the drug of choice in obstruction of the upper airway.

VI.30 Trichlorethylene:
A is incompatible with activated charcoal
B is analgesic at sub-anaesthetic concentrations
C causes deep sighing respiration
D decreases the tone and contractility of the pregnant uterus
E frequently causes ventricular arrhythmias during deep levels
   of anaesthesia.

VI.31 Nitrous oxide:

- A   increases the size of a pneumothorax
- B   induces bone marrow aplasia following prolonged exposure
- C   was first prepared by Priestley in 1864
- D   is relatively insoluble in blood
- E   is 10 times more soluble in fat than in blood.

VI.32 Evidence for the existence of drug receptors includes:

- A   some drugs act at great dilution
- B   access to the site of action is faster than could be explained by diffusion alone
- C   concentration of drugs occurs at special regions of cell membranes
- D   active drugs have a specific stereochemistry
- E   a plot of dose against response is not linear.

VI.33 Inherited enzyme defects modify the response to:

- A   dicoumarol
- B   succinylcholine
- C   tetracycline
- D   atracurium
- E   thiopentone.

VI.34 Hartmann's solution contains

- A   150 mmol sodium
- B   111 mmol chloride
- C   5 mmol potassium
- D   29 mmol lactate in place of bicarbonate
- E   0.5 mmol calcium.

VI.35 Lignocaine:

- A   is completely metabolised by first pass effect if taken orally
- B   lasts longer than procaine
- C   causes local vasodilatation
- D   is absorbed from mucous membranes
- E   causes cerebral depression in overdose.

VI.36 Bupivacaine

- A is an amide
- B produces local vasoconstriction
- C maximum safe dose is 2 mg/kg
- D produces myocardial depression
- E deteriorates on re-autoclaving.

VI.37 Dantrolene:

- A is a muscle relaxant
- B aborts the symptoms of malignant hyperpyrexia in susceptible swine
- C produces severe myocardial depression
- D is only slightly soluble in water
- E hypersensitivity is a risk.

VI.38 The following statements are true:

- A aspirin is absorbed best in the ionised form
- B indomethacin can cause bleeding from any point in the gastro-intestinal tract
- C paracetamol given chronically can cause renal damage
- D soluble aspirin tablets form calcium acetylsalicylate in water
- E phenacetin is addictive.

VI.39 Morphine:

- A crosses the placental barrier
- B does not affect the uterus during labour
- C causes spasm of the sphincter of Oddi, which is relieved by atropine
- D should be administered with care in patients with myotonia
- E decreases plasma ADH concentrations.

VI.40 Histamine release has been reported following administration of:

- A thiopentone
- B atracurium
- C morphine
- D d-tubocurarine
- E etomidate.

VI.41 **The accuracy of blood pressure measurement with the oscillotonometer:**
  A   is dependent upon the velocity of blood flow in the upper arm
  B   is satisfactory down to a systolic pressure of 50 mm Hg
  C   may be affected by pulse rate
  D   suggests that mean blood pressure correlates best with maximum needle deflection
  E   is improved by a slow cuff deflation rate.

VI.42 **Central venous pressure measurement:**
  A   should always be carried out with the patient supine
  B   should be zeroed at the sterno-manubrial angle
  C   gives normal values of right atrial pressure that should not exceed +10 cms water
  D   requires a catheter placed in the right atrium
  E   can be accurately measured with an arterial pressure transducer.

VI.43 **In the measurement of lung compliance:**
  A   airway pressure is zero at the end-expiratory volume, which equals functional fesidual capacity
  B   airway pressure is related to lung volume to construct a pressure-volume curve
  C   on either side of the airway zero pressure point on the curve, the relationship between presssure and volume is linear, and the slope of the line gives a measurement of combined lung and thoracic compliance
  D   normal lung compliance is approximately 0.5 L/cm water
  E   lung compliance alone can be measured by recording the static transpulmonary pressure using an oesophageal balloon.

VI.44 **Measurement of body fluid spaces:**
  A   indocyanine green is excreted unchanged in the urine
  B   extracellular fluid volume is measured using deuterium or tritium
  C   intracellular fluid volume is measured indirectly from extracellular volume and total body water
  D   plasma volume is measured with radio iodinated serum albumin
  E   chromium labelled red cells may be used to measure blood volume.

VI.45 **Statistics:**
  A   in a Gaussian distribution 68% of values lie within +/− one standard error of the mean
  B   Student's 't' test is so called because it is for beginners in statistics
  C   the Chi squared test is used to compare frequencies
  D   if $p < 0.01$ then an observation is significant and there is no possibility that it could have occurred by chance
  E   the sum of the observations divided by the number is the median value.

VI.46 Induction of anaesthesia with a volatile agent:

A is slower if the cardiac output is low
B is quicker if the alveolar ventilation is high
C depends directly on the saturated vapour pressure of the agent
D can be speeded up by adding carbon dioxide to the inspired gases
E is faster in children than in adults.

VI.47 Regarding pH and ionic dissociation:

A a weak acid will be 1000 times more ionised at a pH of 7 than at pH of 4
B a strong alkali will have a high pK
C the pH is inversely proportional to the hydrogen ion concentration
D a pH of 7.7 corresponds to a hydrogen ion concentration of 20 nmols/l
E in the adult there is a hundred fold range of H^+ concentration that is compatible with life.

VI.48 Osmotic diuresis:

A can be achieved with 10 ml/kg of 10% mannitol
B may result in rebound cerebral oedema
C ideally should be with a substance of low molecular weight
D the substance should be rapidly metabolised to limit its action
E occurs with hyperglycaemia.

VI.49 Tissue fluids:

A the normal lymph flow is 2–4 litres/24 hours
B hydrostatic pressure at the arterial end of the capillary is approximately 20 mm Hg
C normal plasma protein oncotic pressure is 25 mm Hg
D with the exception of plasma protein, extravascular, extracellular fluid is identical to plasma
E the renal molecular threshold is approximately 75,000.

VI.50 Surgical diathermy:

A uses a frequency measured in MHz
B may interfere with a demand pacemaker
C the total current flowing through the tips of the diathermy forceps is far more than that flowing through the plate
D the device must not be earthed, to prevent earth loops and the risk of 'microshock'
E works on the same principle as cautery, but is less likely to cause explosions with inflammable gases.

VI.51 Normal laboratory values include:
- **A** serum bicarbonate 24–32 mmol/L
- **B** serum albumin 35–50 grams/L
- **C** creatinine clearance 40–75 ml/min/m^2
- **D** serum magnesium 0.07–0.09 mmol/L
- **E** creatinine 45–125 mmol/L.

VI.52 The Fluotec Mark 3 halothane vaporiser:
- **A** is only accurate at fresh gas flows in excess of 1.5 litres/min
- **B** is susceptible to back pressure effects
- **C** can only be used with halothane
- **D** should be positioned on the upstream side of a trichoroethylene vaporiser on the Boyle's machine
- **E** should be serviced at five yearly intervals.

VI.53 Considering sterilisation:
- **A** moist heat, ie boiling for 15 mins kills bacteria but not spores.
- **B** chemical sterilisation works by coagulation or alkylation of proteins
- **C** ethylene oxide sterilisation requires exposure to a 10% concentration for seven days
- **D** at least 4 hours flushing with air is necessary to clear a ventilator after ethylene oxide sterilisation
- **E** gamma irradiation is unsuitable for endotracheal tubes.

VI.54 Concerning the venturi and choanda effects:
- **A** the venturi effect can be used to enrich or dilute the oxygen content of inspired air
- **B** the entrainment ratio is equal to the entrained flow divided by the driving flow
- **C** the choanda effect results in differential gas or blood flow in the two limbs of a bifurcation associated with a constriction
- **D** the choanda effect only occurs in association with a venturi
- **E** a combination of choanda and venturi effects provides a suitable valve mechanism for artificial ventilation.

VI.55 The following are true:
- **A** Boyle's law states that at constant pressure the volume of a given gas is inversely proportional to its absolute temperature
- **B** Boyle's law states that at constant temperature the pressure of a given mass of gas is inversely proportional to its volume
- **C** Charles' law states that the volume of a given mass of gas at constant pressure is directly proportional to its absolute temperature
- **D** Dalton's law states that the combined pressure of a mixture of gases is equal to the sum of the partial pressures of the constituent gases
- **E** Avogadro's hypothesis states that at constant volume and temperature one gram molecule of any gas exerts the same pressure.

VI.56 Nitrous oxide:

A   the filling ratio of a nitrous oxide cylinder is 0.69
B   1000 gallons of nitrous oxide weigh 30 oz
C   boiling point is $-89\,°C$
D   is unaffected by soda-lime
E   will support combustion of flammable agents in the absence of oxygen.

VI.57 The PaCO$_2$ can be readily determined with:

A   a Severinghaus electrode
B   a Clark electrode
C   the Astrup technique
D   Riley analysis
E   gas chromatography.

VI.58 These are true in the SI system of measurement:

A   the basic unit of mass is the gram
B   pico is the prefix denoting 10^{-12}
C   the Hertz is the derived unit of frequency
D   it is still allowable to use temperature on the centigrade (Celsius) scale
E   the units of resistance to fluid flow are $kg\ m^{-4}\ s^{-3}$.

VI.59 Concerning heat:

A   specific heat capacity is the amount of heat required to raise the temperature of 1 kg of a substance by 1 Kelvin degree
B   heat capacity is the amount of heat required to raise the temperature of a given object by 1 Kelvin degree
C   latent heat is that required to change the state of a substance without change in temperature
D   the freezing seen on the outside of a nitrous oxide cylinder is a result of the latent heat of vaporisation
E   volatile anaesthetics gain heat when they are vaporised.

VI.60 Concerning temperature:

A   1 Kelvin is 1/273.16 of the thermodynamic temperature of the triple point of water
B   the triple point of water occurs at $-0.05°C$
C   alcohol thermometers are unsuitable for high temperatures because alcohol boils at $55°C$
D   mercury solidifies at $-39°C$
E   more than two minutes are necessary for thermal equilibration to be achieved with a mercury thermometer.

VI.1 TFFFF

A Dopamine is released at synapses from interneurones.
B Metacholine is a synthetic beta-methyl analogue of ACh.
C,D,E GABA = gamma-amino butyric acid. 5-HT = 5-hydroxytryptamine.

Glycine is an amino-acid. All have been described at various synapses in the CNS but none at autonomic ganglia.

VI.2 TFTFF

A,D LDH catalyses the interconversion of lactate and pyruvate, the co-enzyme(NAD: nicotinamide adenine dinucleotide) accepting the hydrogen from lactate.
B,E Hydrolysis is the splitting of a molecule with water as one of the reactants. Lactose, a disaccharride, is hydrolysed by lactase to galactose and glucose.

VI.3 TFFTT

B Uptake is in the proximal small bowel.
C Steroids lower plasma $[Ca^{2+}]$, and deplete the bone matrix, ie the organic material.

VI.4 FTTFF

A Correct figure, but cells are NEGATIVE inside.
B Potassium is the major intracellular cation.
D Repolarisation occurs by changes in permeability, not changes in ionic concentrations.

VI.5 FFTFF

A,B,D,E Critical closing pressure is the intraluminal pressure in a capillary which is insufficient to maintain flow and therefore allows the vessel to collapse. It may be contributed to by the activity of precapillary sphincters or by external forces, but neither are the sole determinants.

VI.6   TTTTF

E They are inhibited by Golgi tendon organ feedback, but via Ib afferents, not Ia.

VI.7   TTFTF

C,D Only histamine.

VI.8   TTFFF

C It is a very important factor in the release of energy from FFA and increases the plasma concentration, though it takes some hours. FFA provide a good source of energy in hypoglycaemia, fasting and stress.

D True for monkey and human GH, but not so for a wider range of species.

E Only some of its effects, not, for instance, its effects on carbohydrate metabolism.

VI.9   TTTFT

B Probably best true since aldosterone causes water retention – aldosterone levels are only marginally raised by anaesthetic and operative stress.

D Cortisol if anything produces a mild diuresis.

VI.10   TTTFF

A,C Pure parietal cell secretion is probably isotonic hydrochloric acid: The ph will be less than 1

D Vagotomy will not abolish secretion regulated by local influences.

E This is true for gastric acid and gastrin but secretin has no effect on acid secretion and cannot be part of this loop.

VI.11 TTFTF

C,E   Stimulation – inhibition is the way in which anti-platelet drugs such as aspirin and dipyrimadole act

VI.12 TTTFT

D   Not always: concentrations are elevated when a subject is chronically exposed to antigens, eg during the hay fever season.

VI.13 TTFFF

C   The pathway decussates after the nuclei.
D   The abolition of pain would be far easier if this were true.
E   Referred pain cannot be said to be "conducted" in the same way as a somatic afferent from a specific site.

VI.14 TTFFF

D   Although highly active, its very high blood flow means that the A-V oxygen difference is only ♦ 4 ml.
E   Changes in the renal vascular resistance alter renal blood flow and thus GFR cannot be independent of resistance.

VI.15 TTTFT

D   75%

VI.16 TTTTF

A,B,C Gases in general are more soluble in liquids at lower temperatures.
As a separate phenomenon the affinity of haemoglobin for oxygen is increased.

E   Blood viscosity is INCREASED in hypothermia.

VI.17 FTTTT

A   The concentration is constant, the partial pressure falls.
D   Hyperventilation, caused by hypoxia, reduces $PaCO_2$.

VI.18 TFTTT

B   Increases during controlled ventilation.

VI.19 TTTFF

Draw the curve first.

A   Adult Hb has a lower affinity.
E   Passage through the lungs lowers the CO_2 and raises the pH: the curve shifts to the left.

VI.20 FFFFF

Compliance is the ease with which the thorax distends to a pressure change ("volume per pressure"). It must therefore be greater when the lungs are less full (**B,C**) provided that there is no massive airway collapse. It can be measured either as static or dynamic compliance, breathing spontaneously or with IPPV (**A**).

D   It is always a function of both lung and chest wall compliance.
E   200 ml/cm H_2O.

VI.21 FTFTT
- **B**   The pulse often slows with average clinical doses, presumably due to central vagal action; it is rarely marked, and is usually absent after rapid intravenous injection.
- **C**   This is negligible in humans.

VI.22 TFTFF
- **B**   Dopaminergic stimulation except in high doses. The question asks for PRIMARY mode of action.
- **D**   Mainly beta, mild alpha.
- **E**   Alpha and beta, direct and indirect sympathomimetic amine.

VI.23 FTFTF
- **A**   Direct and indirect.
- **C**   Alpha and beta.
- **E**   Indicated in cases of hypotension due to overdose of ganglion blockers.

VI.24 TFTTF
- **B**   Clonidine has rather different actions if given acutely or chronically. It is certainly a partial alpha agonist but its most important anti-hypertensive action is on alpha receptors in the CNS.
- **C**   Intravenous administration can cause initial vasoconstriction (alpha).
- **E**   Total daily dose is 200 micrograms to 2 milligrams.

VI.25 TTTTF
- **C**   True: affecting production of factors dependent on vitamin K, ie II (prothrombin), VII, IX and X
- **E**   Doesn't interfere with the fibrinolytic cascade.

VI.26 TTFTF

C   Intracranial pressure is not increased provided that the patient is ventilated, preventing any rise in $PaCO_2$

D   True, if vasodilators are given before the cranium is opened.

E   Etomidate sedation reduces raised intracranial pressure.

VI.27 FTTFF

A   Ammonium chloride.

D   This is used to treat metabolic alkalosis.

E   Kidneys conserve hydrogen ions to compensate.

VI.28 TTFTF

C   Tricyclic antidepressant.

E   Phenothiazine used in the treatment of schizophrenia and related psychoses.

VI.29 TTFTF

A,C It is reasonable to expect that you should know something of the general formulae of the barbiturates and you will find it in any good textbook of pharmacology.

E   Inhalational anaesthesia is the method of choice.

VI.30 FTFFT

A   The interaction is with soda-lime.

C   Rapid, shallow respiration.

D   Unlike halothane.

VI.31 TTFTF
- **C** It was Priestley, but in 1772 – it was introduced into anaesthesia in 1844.
- **E** No, oil/water solubility coefficient 3.2.

VI.32 TFTTF
One of the major topics of general pharmacology and one that you should read about in some detail.
- **B** Ease of passing membranes has nothing to do with subsequent mode of action.

VI.33 FTFFT
- **A** Effects are modified by alterations in, or competition for, plasma protein binding, but these are not inherited.
- **B** Pseudocholinesterase deficiency.
- **C** Not reported.
- **D** Abnormalities of Hoffman degradation have not been reported.
- **E** Porphyria.

VI.34 FTTTF
- **A** 131 mmol sodium
- **E** 2 mmol calcium.

VI.35 FTTTF
- **A** Lignocaine is well absorbed but two thirds is removed by first pass elimination and hence plasma concentrations are low and unpredictable.
- **E** A massive overdose will cause cerebral depression but the clinical answer is that it causes convulsions.

VI.36 TFTTT
B   Produces mild vasodilation.
E   Should certainly not be re-autoclaved more than once.

VI.37 TTFTF
C   Dantrolene is only a mild myocardial depressant.
D   It is much more soluble in alkaline solution.
E   Hypersensitivity has not been demonstrated.

VI.38 FTTTF
A   Drugs are usually best absorbed in the unionised lipid-soluble form.
C   It is possible that prolonged chronic use of any of the anti-pyretic analgesics may have the propensity to cause renal damage. If the option were worded, "paracetamol causes renal damage', it would be far harder to give a definite answer.
D   The tablets are aspirin + citric acid + calcium carbonate.
E   The story of phenacetin "addiction" in a town in Sweden is interesting, but phenacetin is not pharmacologically addictive.

VI.39 TTFTF
C   Careful! – yes it does cause sphincteric spasm, but this isn't relieved by atropine.
E   Increases them directly, though postoperatively may reduce abnormally elevated levels secondary to producing pain relief.

VI.40 TTTTT
E   Recent reports indicate low incidence but it does occur.

VI.41 TFTTT

B Inaccurate below 70 – 80 mm Hg.
C Inaccurate in patients with irregular rhythms, eg atrial fibrillation.

VI.42 FFTFT

A Any position can be used provided it is kept constant.
B This may be a convenient zero to use but is above the right atrium when supine. It doesn't matter where zero is as long as it is kept constant and allowance is made for the verical distance from the atrium.
C True probably, although we are not told from where the zero is measured.
D Anywhere in the chest will do – there must not be any valves between the catheter tip and the right atrium.
E True – no transducer is specific for any particular measurement – it just needs recalibrating (spanning) for lower pressures.

VI.43 TTTFT

A Strictly, airway pressure is atmospheric.
D Normal lung compliance alone is 0.22 L/cm water.

VI.44 FFTTT

A Patients don't have green urine after cardiac output measurements!
B These are used to measure total body water.
E True, provided the haematocrit is also measured.

VI.45 FFTFF

A Gaussian = normal, so 68% is the correct figure but in relation to the standard DEVIATION. The standard ERROR allows an estimate of the true position of the mean.
B It is named after the man who described the distribution: he published the work under the pseudonym "Student".
D If you answered TRUE then you have a poor understanding of the rudiments of statistics and should seek help. Briefly: STATISTICAL significance does not mean REAL (eg clinical) significance, and there is ALWAYS a possibility that things could have occurred by chance (that is what $p < 0.01$ means).
E This is the definition of the mean. Median = middlemost (and equals the mean for a normal distribution).

VI.46 FTFTF

If you marked **A** and **B** incorrectly you lack the basic ideas of the uptake of volatile agents. Go to the standard textbooks, and ask for tutorial help.

C   Not directly, although the relation of SVP, MAC and maximum overpressure can affect induction.

E   Cardiac output is relatively higher than minute ventilation in a child.

VI.47 TTFTF

An understanding of logarithms and pH units will explain these answers but a full consideration is outside the scope of this book.

A   3 pH units = 1000 times.

B   ie it is able to ionise even in highly alkaline solutions.

C   It is a logarithmic relation, not a simple inverse one.

E   6.8 to 7.8 is 1 pH unit, which is tenfold.

VI.48 TTTFT

B   The mannitol that crosses into the brain cells "holds" the water there after the systemic loss of fluid with the amnnitol through the kidneys.

D   Osmotic diuretics depend on not being metabolised.

VI.49 TFTTF

B   35 mm Hg

E   69,000

VI.50 TTFFF

B   A complex subject: the pacemaker may "see" the diathermy as an R wave and fail to pace.

C   The total current flowing in an electrical circuit is constant; this will be true for diathermy unless a fault develops allowing parallel current flow to earth.

D   Earth loops and microshock are not caused simply by earthing: read about this.

E   Cautery is direct burning of tissue by heating of the electrode. Diathermy is a higher energy source than cautery.

VI.51 TTTFF
- **D**   Too low by a factor of 10:0.7–0.9 mmol/L.
- **E**   Wrong units, right figures: micromols/L.

VI.52 FFFFF
- **A**   Accurate down to low flows (Mark 3).
- **B**   Long inlet tube minimises this effect.
- **C**   Only ACCURATE with halothane.
- **D**   Downstream – volatile liquid with the highest boiling point first.
- **E**   Annual servicing recommended.

VI.53 TTFTF
- **C**   8 – 12 hours.
- **E**   Often the method of choice.

VI.54 TTTTT

VI.55 FTTTF

You must know the gas laws. Remember the wording can be confusing when you are in the examination hall.
- **B**   Boyle: pressure and volume.
- **E**   This follows from the hypothesis (equal volumes contain equal numbers of molecules) but is not a statement of it.

VI.56 TFTTT

    B   Wrong by a factor of 10 (a catch often used) – 100 galls.

    E   Above 450°C decomposition will produce a 33% oxygen mixture.

VI.57 TFTTF

    B   Is an oxygen electrode.

    E   Measures gas content in gaseous not blood phase.

VI.58 FTTTT

    A   The unit of mass is the kilogram.

    E   You should be able to work this out from the Hagen-Poiseuille formula.

VI.59 TTTTF

    E   They lose heat during vaporisation (as in **D**) and vaporisers are designed to minimise this.

VI.60 TFFTT

    B   Triple point of water is +0.01°C

    C   Alcohol boils at 78.5°C

Paper VII   Questions

VII.1 Adrenaline:
- **A** is synthesised from nor-adrenaline by a methyl transferase in the adrenal medulla and nerve endings
- **B** increases the basal metabolic rate
- **C** is metabolised in the liver
- **D** stimulates glycogenolysis
- **E** causes systolic and diastolic hypertension when injected intravenously.

VII.2 Glucose:
- **A** the normal fasting concentration is about 4 mmol/L
- **B** is converted into glucose-1-phosphate by the action of hexokinase
- **C** is converted into glycogen in both skeletal muscle and liver
- **D** is produced enzymically from glycogen in skeletal muscle and liver
- **E** has about the same concentration in plasma and glomerular filtrate.

VII.3 The chief factors controlling sodium excretion are:
- **A** hydrostatic pressure in peritubular capillaries
- **B** rate of tubular secretion of H^+ and K^+
- **C** aldosterone
- **D** vasa recta blood flow
- **E** blood pH.

VII.4 Cerebral blood flow is raised by:
- **A** hypercarbia
- **B** the head down position
- **C** inhalational anaesthetic agents
- **D** sitting up
- **E** sodium nitroprusside.

VII.5 Pacemaker activity in the myocardium:
- **A** is not abnormal in Purkinje fibres
- **B** is normal in isolated ventricular tissue in vitro
- **C** its onset coincides with the start of systole
- **D** in the sino-atrial node, starts from a maximum repolarisation to a value less negative than in other cardiac cells
- **E** is not slowed by temperature, bradycardia then results from the threshold to the action potential being increased.

VII.6   Muscle spindles:

    A   are receptors which excite the normal reflex arc

    B   afferent impulses are carried by fusimotor fibres

    C   respond to a rise in muscle tension either from contraction or external stretch

    D   are bundles of modified intrafusal fibres equipped with sensory nerve endings

    E   are structures which indicate a change in muscle length.

VII.7   Both angiotensin and serotinin:

    A   are formed by proteolysis

    B   cause constriction of skin blood vessels

    C   cause the release of aldosterone

    D   are present in entero-chromaffin cells

    E   are amines.

VII.8   The secretion of growth hormone is stimulated by:

    A   hypoglycaemia

    B   anaesthesia

    C   cortisol

    D   rapid-eye-movement sleep

    E   dopamine receptor agonists.

VII.9   The membrane potential of a nerve fibre:

    A   represents an imbalance of negative to positive ions on the two sides of a semi-permeable membrane

    B   can be calculated from the Nernst equation

    C   is inversely related to the diameter of the fibre

    D   is measured, conventionally, as negative on the inside

    E   reverses its polarity during an action potential.

VII.10   Bile:

    A   secretion is increased by cholecystokinin

    B   is made more acidic in the gall bladder

    C   is concentrated up to forty-fold in the gall bladder

    D   contains bilirubin that is mainly unconjugated

    E   is secreted by the parenchymal cells of the liver.

VII.11 Normal coagulation mechanisms in vivo:

  A the intrinsic pathway is activated through exposure to electronegatively charged wettable surfaces
  B intrinsic pathway activation involves factors XI and XII
  C thrombin is a proteolytic enzyme
  D extrinsic pathway activation involves tissue thromboplastin (factor V)
  E thrombin increases platelet aggregation.

VII.12 Hypersensitivity:

  A type 1 immediate hypersensitivity involves IgE
  B antigen excess in type 3 produces an Arthus response
  C delayed hypersensitivity is cell-mediated
  D type 2 hypersensitivity binds complement
  E cell-mediated hypersensitivity involves complement.

VII.13 The electroencepholagram:

  A is depressed by anaesthetics in a specific predictable manner
  B is a measure of summed evoked cortical potentials
  C the alpha rhythm is the dominant rhythm in the alert conscious subject
  D the delta rhythm is associated with rapid eye movement sleep
  E the alpha rhythm frequency is decreased by high $PaCO_2$.

VII.14 In the glomerulus:

  A the colloid osmotic pressure is higher in the efferent than in the afferent arterioles
  B the filtration pressure is the difference between the hydrostatic pressures in Bowman's capsule and the tubule
  C molecules up to molecular weight 5000 are filtered freely
  D molecules of molecular weight over 50,000 are not filtered at all
  E GFR = concentration in the urine multiplied by the plasma concentration divided by the urine volume.

VII.15 Water excretion:

  A the ascending limb of the Loop of Henle is impermeable to water
  B sodium reabsorption from the Loop of Henle occurs passively
  C under conditions of maximum antidiuresis, 5% of water reabsorption occurs in the distal tubule
  D anuria is defined as a urine output of less than 0.1 ml/kg/hour
  E prolonged thirst induces aldosterone production.

VII.16 When calculating the dead space using the Bohr equation:

A   arterial or end-tidal samples to estimate the CO_2 are
     equivalent
B   there must be a steady-state
C   the assumption is of two "fractions" in each tidal volume
D   the result is equivalent to a volume of each breath that takes
     no part in gas exchange
E   the result is usually expressed at STPD.

VII.17 Voluntary hyperventilation for three minutes:

A   raises arterial CO_2 tension
B   causes facial paraesthesiae
C   causes cerebral hypoxia
D   decreases arterial O_2 tension
E   may result afterwards in periodic ventilation.

VII.18 Anatomical dead space:

A   increases with increasing age
B   increases in the sitting position
C   decreases with extension of the neck
D   is approximately 10 ml/Kg body weight in an adult male
E   is reduced by nasotracheal intubation.

VII.19 The capacity of haemoglobin for oxygen:

A   is decreased by temperature
B   is decreased by 2,3-diphosphoglycerate
C   under normal conditions is about 1.35 mls oxygen per gram
     of haemoglobin
D   is reduced by increased $PaCO_2$
E   is reduced by carbon monoxide.

VII.20 Intrapleural pressure:

A   in quiet respiration is 3–10 cm H_2O below atmospheric
     pressure
B   varies during the respiratory cycle
C   is uninfluenced by PEEP
D   is 30–55 cm H_2O above atmospheric pressure on deep
     inspiration
E   is always negative.

VII.21 Atropine and hyoscine:
- **A** increase the risk of regurgitation
- **B** are contra-indicated in glaucoma
- **C** in large doses cause mild neuromuscular blockade
- **D** are equipotent as drying agents
- **E** are both CNS stimulants.

VII.22 Vasoconstrictor drugs which exert little or no positive inotropic effect include:
- **A** adrenaline
- **B** methoxamine
- **C** isoprenaline
- **D** dobutamine
- **E** metaraminol.

VII.23 Phenoxybenzamine:
- **A** sedation and fatigue are side-effects
- **B** forms a non-dissociating bond with the alpha adrenergic receptor
- **C** may precipitate adrenaline-induced arrhythmias
- **D** block cannot be reversed pharmacologically
- **E** initial central stimulation may cause vomiting.

VII.24 Alpha-methyldopa:
- **A** oral dosage is 0.5 to 3 gm daily
- **B** causes a negative sodium balance
- **C** causes hepatocellular jaundice
- **D** results in the formation of a false neurotransmitter
- **E** sedation is a very common side-effect.

VII.25 Protamine:
- **A** is a basic protein
- **B** 1 mg antagonises 100 mg heparin
- **C** is a myocardial stimulant
- **D** is contraindicated in hepatic failure
- **E** is 60% protein bound.

VII.26 Central sedation is produced by:

    A hyoscine

    B prochlorperazine

    C diphenhydramine

    D atropine

    E doxapram.

VII.27 Hypokalaemia is produced by:

    A triamterene

    B carbenoxolone sodium

    C frusemide

    D spironolactone

    E ammonium chloride.

VII.28 Prednisolone is preferred to hydrocortisone in the treatment of inflammation because:

    A it causes less gastric irritation

    B it causes less sodium retention

    C it does not suppress the secretion of corticotrophin

    D it has no effect on gluconeogenesis

    E it is available orally.

VII.29 Halothane:

    A has a saturated vapour pressure of approximately one third of a standard atmosphere

    B depresses the blood pressure mainly by its direct action on beta-adrenergic receptors

    C does not cause respiratory depression until stage III of surgical anaesthesia

    D sensitizes the myocardium to catecholamines

    E should not be used in any jaundiced patients.

VII.30 Barbiturates:

    A were introduced by Fischer and von Mehring in 1940

    B are readily taken up into body fat

    C the long acting drugs (e.g. phenobarbitone) are excreted unchanged in the urine

    D distribution in the body is influenced by blood pH

    E hepatic metabolism is largely responsible for the breakdown of the ultra-short acting drugs (e.g. thiopentone).

VII.31 Isoflurane and enflurane:

  A have similar boiling points
  B have similar molecular weights
  C are contra-indicated in anephric patients
  D adrenaline infiltration is relatively safe
  E both give measurable fluoride ion in the serum.

VII.32 The following local anaesthetic agents are broken down by pseudocholinesterase:

  A lignocaine
  B procaine
  C amethocaine — tetracaine
  D cinchocaine
  E bupivacaine.

VII.33 The following pairs of drugs have synergistic effects:

  A penicillin and tetracycline
  B penicillin and streptomycin
  C reserpine and chlorothiazide
  D tolbutamide and sulphadimidine
  E atracurium and gentamicin.

VII.34 Intravenous fluids

  A "dextrose-saline" is 0.18% saline in 5% dextrose
  B 1 litre of "dextrose-saline" contains 31 mmol sodium
  C the normal urine sodium excretion per 24 hours varies between 70 and 150 mmol
  D the normal urine potassium excretion per 24 hours is approximately 70 mmol
  E the calorie yield from 1 litre of 20% glucose is 800 kCal.

VII.35 Cocaine:

  A causes local anaesthesia by blocking synaptic transmission
  B potentiates the effects of exogenous catecholamines
  C is partially hydrolysed by cholinesterase
  D the toxic dose is 500 mgm 100 mg
  E causes mydriasis.

VII.36 Characteristics of neuromuscular blockade by non-depolarising relaxants include:

 A   progressive diminution of the duration of the end-plate potential

 B   lowered end-plate potential amplitude for a given quantal release of acetylcholine

 C   ganglion blockade

 D   post tetanic facilitation

 E   hypertonus if the patient has myotonia.

VII.37 Plasma cholinesterase activity affects the duration of action of:

 A   propanidid

 B   edrophonium

 C   atracurium

 D   suxamethonium

 E   procaine.

VII.38 Morphine:

 A   is metabolised by the liver

 B   causes a lowering of the $PaCO_2$

 C   can be reversed by naloxone

 D   causes diarrhoea

 E   causes miosis.

VII.39 The following drugs cause diarrhoea:

 A   codeine

 B   neostigmine

 C   atropine

 D   pethidine

 E   carbenoxolone.

VII.40 Retroperitoneal fibrosis is a side-effect of treatment with:

 A   methylpentynol

 B   ethosuximide

 C   methysergide

 D   practolol

 E   prednisolone.

VII.41 Manometers:

A a pressure which supports a 7.5 mm column of mercury will support a 10.2 cm column of water

B 1 kPa is equal to a pressure of 7.5 mm mercury

C a mercury column used in a sphygmomanometer is closed at the top to prevent contamination and spillage

D a mercury barometer used to measure atmospheric pressure is sealed with a vacuum above the surface of the liquid

E aneroid gauges do not contain liquid.

VII.42 Oxygen saturation measurement:

A spectrophotometric estimation depends upon the quantity of reduced haemoglobin

B at the isobestic point, light absorption is equal for both oxy-and reduced haemoglobin

C measurement at the isobestic point provides a reference point independent of haemoglobin concentration

D oxygen content measurements can be made on whole blood

E carbon monoxide interferes with normal oximeter readings.

VII.43 The Wright peak flow meter:

A is a variable orifice flowmeter

B rotation of the vane opens up a slot for venting of expired gas

C the rate and number of rotations of the vane is proportional to peak flow

D the peak flow of a fit adult male is 500 L/min or more

E the subject is allowed three attempts at the instrument, the first of which is ignored.

VII.44 When using a flow-directed, balloon-tipped, pulmonary artery catheter (Swan-Ganz):

A one obtains a direct measurement of the left atrial pressure

B once in situ the balloon should be left inflated to prevent displacement

C 'wedge' pressure is approximately equal to the left ventricular end-diastolic pressure in the normal, fit adult

D the volume of the balloon is 5 ml

E pressures should be measured at end-expiration.

VII.45 Randomisation of two treatments in a clinical trial means that:

A results are treated in random order

B treatments are chosen in relation to some predictable event

C results are analysed by Student's t-test

D treatments can be allocated by reference to series of random numbers

E treatments are chosen by an independent person.

VII.46 When considering the uptake of a volatile anaesthetic agent:

   A   the rate of uptake is increased if ventilation increases
   B   induction is more rapid if cardiac output falls
   C   induction is less rapid with a less soluble agent
   D   the effect of changing cardiac output on the rate of uptake
       will be far greater with a more soluble agent
   E   the second-gas effect allows the maintenance concentration
       of halothane to be reduced when nitrous oxide is used.

VII.47 A consideration of acid-base balance:

   A   the buffering power of plasma is greater in vivo than in vitro
   B   buffering is greater if the haemoglobin concentration is
       higher
   C   base excess will vary with haemoglobin concentration
   D   the normal buffer base is 48 mEq/L
   E   the slope of the buffer line increases as buffering decreases.

**VII.48 The following measurements are consistent with physiological
         oliguria:**

   A   urine sodium <10 mmol/L
   B   urine specific gravity >1.024
   C   urine/plasma osmolality ratio 5:1
   D   urine/plasma urea 100:1
   E   urine/plasma creatinine 20:1.

VII.49 When recording the electrocardiogram:

   A   the amplitude is usually of the order of millivolts
   B   needle electrodes are safer than plate electrodes
   C   mains interference can be reduced by a screened lead
   D   artefacts caused by muscular tremor can be reduced by a
       screened lead
   E   the recorded potential is the sum of the individual
       intracellular action potentials.

VII.50 Normal electrolyte concentrations in body secretions include:

   A   potassium in gastric juice 15 mmol/L
   B   sodium in bile 30 mmol/L
   C   sodium in saliva 112 mmol/L
   D   chloride in gastric juice 140 mmol/L
   E   bicarbonate in pancreatic juice 10 mmol/L.

VII.51 Vaporisers:

- **A** the Boyle's bottle is a plenum vaporiser
- **B** Boyle's bottle has a poor thermal conductivity
- **C** back-pressure on a plenum vaporiser may decrease the concentration of vapour in the gas mixture
- **D** draw-over vaporisers must have a lower internal resistance than plenum types
- **E** the copper kettle is a draw-over vaporiser.

VII.52 Liquid solutions suitable for sterilisation of endotracheal tubes include:

- **A** chlorhexidine
- **B** hexachlorophene
- **C** phenol
- **D** iodine
- **E** ethyl alcohol.

VII.53 With a vaporiser "in circle', the inspired concentration of anaesthetic vapour:

- **A** is always less than the nominal concentration
- **B** always equals or exceeds the nominal concentration
- **C** is independent of flow
- **D** increases if minute ventilation increases
- **E** increases if fresh gas flow increases.

VII.54 Blood flow:

- **A** can be measured ultrasonically
- **B** cardiac output can be measured non-invasively by the Fick principle
- **C** variable orifice flowmeters are used for liquids as well as gases
- **D** to an organ can be calculated solely from measurements of the washout curve of a radioactive isotope
- **E** turbulent flow results in plasma skimming of blood.

VII.55 Concerning gas analysis:

- **A** the Van Slyke apparatus uses a manometric method
- **B** an infra red analyser can be used for the analysis of CO_2, N_2O, diethyl ether and halothane
- **C** the Narkotest halothane analyser uses ultraviolet absorption from a low pressure mercury lamp
- **D** the Lloyd-Haldane apparatus will measure CO_2 to $+/- 0.05\%$
- **E** the Katharometer chromatograph can be used to analyse blood gas contents of nitrogen, carbon dioxide, nitrous oxide and oxygen.

VII.56 Gas Laws:

- **A** equal volumes of all gases at the same temperature contain the same number of molecules
- **B** Avogadro's number is the number of particles in 1 mole of a substance
- **C** 1 mole of any gas at STP occupies 22.4 litres
- **D** on the content gauge of a gas cylinder at constant temperature, pressure is directly proportional to the amount of gas present
- **E** 42 G nitrous oxide occupies 22.4 litres at STP.

VII.57 Gas chromatography is used for:

- **A** detection of impurities in gases
- **B** determination of solubility of anaesthetic gases
- **C** measurement of inhaled gas concentrations
- **D** calibration of anaesthetic vaporisers
- **E** determination of blood concentrations of anaesthetic gases.

VII.58 If a large bubble is connected to a small bubble:

- **A** the pressure in each will be governed by the law of Laplace
- **B** the small bubble will empty into the larger one
- **C** the addition of a detergent to the system will prevent one bubble emptying into the other
- **D** the critical closing pressure is halved
- **E** the bubbles will equalise in size.

VII.59 Humidity:

- **A** absolute humidity is the mass of water-vapour present in a given volume of air
- **B** relative humidity is the ratio of the mass of water vapour present in a given volume of air to the mass required to saturate the same volume of air at the same temperature
- **C** in a hair hygrometer, as humidity rises, the hair becomes shorter and tighter
- **D** Regnault's hygrometer contains mercury
- **E** relative humidity = SVP at dew point × SVP at ambient temperature.

VII.60 Under normal conditions in the U K. heat loss from the body occurs in the proportion of:

- **A** convection 30%
- **B** radiation 50%
- **C** evaporation 10%
- **D** heating of dry air during respiration 2%
- **E** evaporation of water in the respiratory tract 8%.

Paper VII Answers

VII.1 FTTTF

  A Phenyl-ethanolamine N-methyl transferase is found only in the medulla.

  C As well as at the nerve endings.

  E Classically, because it has both alpha and beta activity, it will cause a rise in systolic pressure and a lesser fall in diastolic pressure. The mean pressure will rise. The actual effect will depend also on the prevailing autonomic tone.

VII.2 TTTFT

  B Hexokinase is present in all tissues. The liver also contains the more specific enzyme, glucokinase.

  D Only the liver has the necessary glucose-6-phosphatase. Otherwise, glycogen is broken down to glucose-1-phosphate by phosphorylase and in muscle this compound is catabolised via the citric acid cycle or Embden-Meyehof path.

  E Almost all will then be reabsorbed under normal circumstances.

VII.3 TTTTF

  E This comes as a secondary effect of **B**, but this is not a CHIEF factor.

VII.4 TTTFF

  A,C These cause cerebral vasodilatation.

  B The Trendelenburg position.

VII.5 TFTFT

  C The pacemaker potential precedes the action potential.

  D The wording here is confusing: SA node = −60 mV, other cells about −90 mV. The SA node cannot strictly be said to have a resting potential.

  E Pacemaker activity is slowed by hypothermia.

VII.6 TFTTT

B   Fusimotor fibres are gamma motor EFFERENTS.

VII.7 FTFFF

A,E   Serotonin is an amine (5-hydroxytryptamine); angiotensin
     is a polypeptide.
C   Only angiotensin.
D   Entero-chromaffin cells in the intestinal mucosa secrete
     serotonin.

VII.8 TTFFT

C,D   Decrease secretion.

VII.9 TFFTT

A   The imbalance is extremely small compared to the total
     number of ions. The imbalance is mainly because K^+
     efflux is not accompanied by a corresponding efflux of the
     protein anions.
B   The membrane potential can be calculated from the
     Goldman field equation which involves K^+, Na^+ & Cl^-. The
     Nernst equation is a general equation for calculating a
     potential for a particular ion. The Gibbs-Donnan effect is
     the effect of non-diffusible protein anions on the
     distribution of diffusible ions.
C   The potential is independent of the diameter.

VII.10 FTFFT

A   Cholecystokinin causes gallbladder contraction; secretin
     increases production of bile.
C   The percentage of solids increases from 2–4% to 10–12%
     after maximal concentration.
D,E   Bilirubin glucuronide, the conjugate, is secreted from the
     liver cells into the bile canaliculi.

VII.11 TTTTT

You should be able to draw a diagram of the coagulation cascade.

VII.12 TFTTF

B Antibody excess localises the antigen/antibody reaction: the Arthus response.

E This is Type 4, delayed hypersensitivity, and does not involve complement.

VII.13 FFFFT

A One of the major problems in anaesthesia is to find a reliable, simple, measurable index of the depth of anaesthesia.

B It is a measure of electrical activity in the outermost layers of the grey matter, probably mostly from dendrites.

C The alpha rhythm is seen at rest, relaxed, and with eyes closed.

D The delta rhythm is large slow waves: REM sleep gives a desynchronised, irregular activity.

VII.14 TFTFF

A Water and small molecules will have been filtered leaving the proteins behind.

B There are 2 active pressures: hydrostatic and colloid osmotic pressure.

C,D There is no absolute cut-off: hindrance to filtration begins above 5000 and the normal kidney should just fail to filter any albumin (69,000).

E GFR= urinary concentration divided by plasma concentration multiplied by urine volume (UV/P)

VII.15 TFFTT

B Active from ascending limb, perhaps under the influence of ADH.

C 15%

VII.16 FTTTF

You must know what the Bohr equation is, the assumptions upon which it is based, and how to derive it.

A   Arterial estimation will give the physiological dead space, end-tidal the anatomical. They are virtually the same in the young fit healthy subject.

C   The 2 fractions are the alveolar and the dead space fractions: in reality there will be mixing.

E   Usually BTPS or ATPS.

VII.17 FTTFT

A,D   Increased alveolar ventilation will LOWER $PaCO_2$ and RAISE PaO_2.

B   A symptom of lowered ionized calcium (tetany).

C   By causing cerebral vasoconstriction.

E   Apnoea caused by hypocapnia, and a fluctuating hypoxic drive between the periods of reduced ventilation.

VII.18 TTFFT

C   Increases.

D   Approximately 2 ml/kg.

VII.19 FFTFF

The capacity is the amount at full saturation and there are no considerations of affinity.

VII.20 TTFFF

C   Cannot be true, especially at high values of PEEP.

D   BELOW atmospheric.

E   It will rise above atmospheric pressure in forced expiration.

VII.21 TFFFF

A By reducing the tone of the cardiac sphincter.
B TOPICAL atropine is contra-indicated. The normal
   intravenous dose, 0.6 mgm, will not precipitate glaucoma.
C Atropine has no effect at skeletal muscle (nicotinic).
D Hyoscine is more potent than atropine.
E Hyoscine is a depressant, but it can produce restlessness
   and excitement in the elderly, especially if they are in pain.

VII.22 FTFFT

A Positive inotrope.
C Mainly beta adrenergic action, but some inotropic effect.
D Selective positive inotrope.

VII.23 TTFTT

A Often quite serious, making patients too sleepy to eat.
C Powerful anti-arrhythmic.

VII.24 TFTTT

B It may cause salt and water retention.
D Its anti-hypertensive action is mainly by false transmitter
   in the CNS.
E Adjectives of frequency can cause problems when trying
   to decide "true or false?": here it is "true".

VII.25 TFFFF

B 1 mg protamine antagonises 1 mg heparin (nominally 100
   units).
C Myocardial depressant.
E Highly ionised; protein binding minimal.

VII.26 TTTFF

C   An anti-histamine.
D   Unlike hyoscine, atropine is a central stimulant.
E   Doxapram is an analeptic.

VII.27 FTTFF

A,D   Aldosterone antagonist – hyperkalaemia.
E   Acidifying diuretic – 2 moles ammonium chloride produce
       1 mole of urea (osmotic diuretic) and 1 mole of H$^+$ ions.

VII.28 FTFFF

Prednisolone does cause less sodium retention than
hydrocortisone **(B)** but otherwise the two steroids are pretty well
equivalent in equi-potent dosage. Hydrocortisone IS available
orally **(C)**. In general, the particular steroid to use can depend as
much on the patient as on the indication for use: it is worth
reading around this subject.

VII.29 TFFTF

A   243 mm Hg: remember the SVP does not change with
       ambient pressure.
B   Mainly on the myocardium, but not via the beta receptors.
C   Respiratory depression is progressive with increasing
       concentration. This is true for all commonly used
       inhalational agents except ether.
E   Do not confuse the jaundice of known cause, in a patient
       who has not had a recent anaesthetic, with the problems
       of repeat halothane anaesthesia.

VII.30 FTTTT

A   Were introduced by Fischer and von Mehring, but in 1903.
C   There is some metabolism but it is very slow, 1% per hour
       for phenobarbitone.
E   For the breakdown of the drugs yes, but not the initial
       recovery. Metabolism is of clinical significance in the
       recovery from methohexitone.

VII.31 TFFTT

    A   Isoflurane 58.5°C, enflurane 56.5°C.

    B   They are structural isomers and thus have the SAME molecular weight.

    C   An anephric patient cannot sustain renal damage.

    E   True, though clinically insignificant for isoflurane.

VII.32 FTTFF

In general, ester-linked agents are broken down by liver and plasma esterases; amide-linked agents are N-demethylated and then hydroysed, with some urinary elimination.

VII.33 TTTTT

    A,B   Different spectra and mode of action.

    C   Both antihypertensives, one acting by noradrenaline depletion, the other by direct vasodilation.

    D   Some sulphonamides have hypoglycaemic properties, eg sulphanilamide.

    E   The combination of an aminoglycoside antibiotic and a non-depolarising neuromuscular blocking drug is synergistic at the neuromuscular junction.

VII.34 FTTTT

    A   Standard dextrose solution is 5%, but the usual dextrose-saline is isosmotic and the dextrose component must be 4%.

VII.35 FTTFT

    A   Like other clinically useful local anaesthetics its action is direct on the transmission of nerve impulses along the axon by blocking sodium channels.

    B   Yes, because it inhibits re-uptake at the sympathetic nerve terminal.

    C   It is also hydrolysed in the liver and 10% is excreted unchanged via the kidney.

    D   100 mgm in a 70 kgm man.

VII.36   TTTTF
  E   Hypertonus may follow the use of depolarising relaxants, but the response to non-depolarisers is normal.

VII.37   TFFTT
  B   Is an anticholinesterase itself.
  C   It is metabolised by Hoffman degradation and ester hydrolysis.

VII.38   TFTFT
  A   Mainly by conjugation.
  B   Respiratory depression: the CO_2 will rise.
  D   Constipation by direct action, contracting smooth muscle.
  E   Pupillary constriction.

VII.39   FTFFF
  A   Constipation.
  B   It is a muscarinic analogue of acetyl choline.
  C   Used as an anti-spasmodic.
  D   Pethidine does not cause constipation, but it does not cause diarrhoea either.
  E   Carbenoxolone is an extract of liquorice but it does not cause diarrhoea.

VII.40   FFTTF
  A   Central depressant.
  B   Anticonvulsant.
  E   No evidence.

VII.41 TTFTT

C   No, they are open, measuring the gauge pressure above atmospheric.

VII.42 TTFTF

A   True – this is the normal principle of the oximeter, depending on the ratio between oxy– and reduced haemoglobin.

C   Absorbance at the isobestic point varies with the haemoglobin concentration.

D   True: whole blood can be used, although blood is usually diluted and haemolysed before measurement.

E   Selection of the particular wavelength of light avoids interference by carbon monoxide.

VII.43 TTFTF

C   The vane does not rotate completely but only partially, opposed by force from a coiled spring

E   The best performance is recorded, some patients are so breathless that they can only manage one decent blow!

VII.44 FFTFT

A   It is an indirect pressure transmitted through the pulmonary capillary bed.

B   If left inflated there is a risk of distal pulmonary infarction. The balloon is NOT an aid to fixation.

D   About 1 ml.

E   At FRC, PEEP or CPAP can make the absolute measurement difficult but for clinical purposes one is usually more interested in changes.

VII.45 FFFTF

A   The TREATMENTS are randomised, as **D**.

C   Randomisation does not require any particular statistical test.

D   Random numbers can be looked up from books of statistical tables, or can be generated from the more advanced hand-held calculators.

VII.46 TTFTF

This is an exceedingly important theoretical topic that you must understand. Read and seek help until you do.
C   More rapid.
E   Second-gas and concentration effects are only of significance in the early induction phase. They are anyway of little practical importance.

VII.47 FTFTF

A   There is less buffering power in vivo because of the diffusion of bicarbonate.
B   Haemoglobin is a very important protein buffer: it has six times the buffering capacity of the plasma proteins.
C,D,E Buffer base includes haemoglobin, base excess is independent of it. The steeper the line, the better the buffering. The Sigaard-Andersen nomogram is useful in understanding this.

VII.48 TTFTF

C   Osmolality ratio 2.5:1.
E   Urine/plasma creatinine $\leqslant 48 < 60:1$.

VII.49 TFTFF

B   Needle electrodes = higher current density = higher likelihood of injury if there is a fault.
D   Screening will have no effect on this source of interference: make sure the patient is comfortable, warm and relaxed.
E   It is only the surface expression of this, and over a small area. The sum of the individual action potentials would be enormous – 100 mV multiplied by the total number of cells in the myocardium!

VII.50 TFTTF

B   Bile is rich in sodium 145 mmol/L.
E   Pancreatic juice is rich in bicarbonate 110 mmol/L.

VII.51 TTFTF

  C   Back-pressure increases output concentration.
  E   It is a plenum type with high thermal conductivity.

VII.52 TFFFT

  B   Antisepsis only.
  C,D   Will produce mucosal ulceration and burns.

VII.53 FTFTF

  A,B   Recirculation means that the actual concentration must at
         least be equal to the nominal concentration.
  C   Flow includes both ventilation (D) and fresh gas (E),
         therefore false.
  E   Fresh gas into the circuit will dilute tha anaesthetic vapour.

VII.54 TTTFF

  D   The volume undergoing washout must also be known.
         Flow is equal to the volume undergoing washout divided
         by the time constant of the washout curve.
  E   Plasma skimming is dependent upon laminar flow
         occurring at the centre of the vessel.

VII.55 TTFTT

  A   Measures blood gas content by extraction, reabsorption
         by reagents, and recording of pressure at constant
         volume.
  B   Infra-red can be used for all gases with more than 2 atoms
         in a molecule. If there are only 2 atoms then they must be
         dissimilar.
  C   Apparatus made by Drager that uses the principle of
         change in length of silicon rubber after absorption of
         vapour.

VII.56 FTTTF

A   Must also be at the same pressure.
D   True, refers to situation when only gas is present.
E   44 is the molecular weight of nitrous oxide.

VII.57 TFTTT

B   Gas not liquid phase measurement.

VII.58 TTFFF

A,B,E Pressure = tension/radius. This applies to bubbles (the tension is the surface tension) and also to tubes such as blood vessels (the tension is that in the smooth muscle and elastic tissue).
C   An ordinary detersent will merely lower the overall surface tension.
D   Critical closing pressure is important in a consideration of the behaviour of small blood vessels and the alveoli: it is, however, out of context here.
E   This option and **B** are mutually exclusive: questions like this should not be in the exam. Make sure you answered logically - **B** and **E** cannot BOTH be right or BOTH be wrong whatever is the correct combination.

VII.59 TTFFF

C   The hair becomes longer.
D   Regnault's hygrometer contains ether.
E   Relative humidity = SVP at dew point / SVP at ambient temperature.

VII.60 TFFTT

B   Radiation accounts for 30%
C   Evaporation accounts for 30%

Paper VIII Questions

VIII.1 Acetylcholine at muscarinic receptors:
  A stimulates adrenaline secretion by the adrenal medulla
  B causes vasodilatation
  C increases bronchial tone
  D increases ureteric tone
  E in larger doses stimulates skeletal muscle.

VIII.2 Adenosine triphosphate:
  A is synthesised when skeletal muscle contracts
  B contains two energy-rich phosphate bonds
  C is an integral part of the flavoprotein-cytochrome system
  D is only produced during the aerobic, not anaerobic, catabolism of glucose
  E is hydrolysed enzymically during the operation of the "sodium pump".

VIII.3 The following are consistent with Starling's law of the heart:
  A an increase in central venous pressure can result in a decrease in peripheral resistance
  B a decrease in left ventricular end-diastolic pressure will lower myocardial work
  C the energy of contraction is a function of the length of the muscle fibre
  D the law can still hold if work is represented by stroke volume or change of ventricular pressure with time (dP/dt)
  E an increased afterload will reduce cardiac output.

VIII.4 In a normal Valsalva manouevre:
  A initially the systolic blood pressure rises
  B there will be an increase in pulse rate during the forced expiration
  C control of the blood pressure and heart rate is dependent on arterial baroreceptors
  D the systolic pressure remains raised during the manoeuvre because of increased peripheral resistance
  E is blocked by beta-adrenergic blockade.

VIII.5 The "blood-brain barrier":
  A anatomically, is at the arachnoid villi
  B is less permeable in the neonate
  C results in the total exclusion of many drugs from the brain
  D results in very low catecholamine levels in the brain and spinal cord
  E is functionally similar to a cell membrane.

VIII.6 Pain:

A   transmission normally occurs in the lateral spinothalamic tracts

B   may be modulated at a spinal level by endorphinergic interneurones

C   is modified at a spinal level by descending fibres from the periaqueductal grey matter of the mid-brain

D   fibres from the frontal cortex inhibit thalamic interpretation of pain

E   surgery of the cerebral cortex is not associated with pain.

VIII.7 Prostaglandins are:

A   not naturally occurring substances

B   used to induce abortion and labour

C   metabolised in the pulmonary circulation

D   modulators of histamine and bradykinin action in pain

E   stored in mast cells.

VIII.8 Vasopressin:

A   is a nonapeptide

B   is important in the normal control of blood pressure

C   is inactive by mouth

D   is bound to neurophysin in the pituitary

E   the threshold to secretion is about 280 mOsm/L.

VIII.9 The normal, non-specialised, cell membrane is:

A   more permeable to sodium than to potassium

B   freely permeable to water

C   of low electrical capacity

D   freely permeable to mannitol

E   more easily penetrated by lipid-soluble than by water-soluble molecules.

VIII.10 The nerve action potential:

A   is initiated by potassium efflux

B   is propogated exponentially

C   transmission is "saltatory" between the nodes of Ranvier

D   conduction is faster in "pain" fibres than "temperature" fibres

E   is approximately 110mV above the resting potential.

VIII.11 Physiological anticlotting mechanisms include:

    A   local liberation of endogenous anticoagulents (eg heparin)
    B   hepatic removal of activated clotting factors
    C   clotting factor consumption
    D   streptokinase liberation
    E   fibrinolytic activation.

VIII.12 Complement:

    A   is primarily responsible for cytolysis
    B   alternative pathway activation requires prior exposure to the antigen
    C   produces immune adherence
    D   activation produces anaphylotoxin C4a
    E   is an acute phase reactant.

VIII.13 The pressure of the cerebrospinal fluid:

    A   is normally approximately 120 mm Hg in the lateral level position
    B   fluctuates with the blood pressure
    C   is unaffected by quiet breathing
    D   is raised by Queckenstedt's test
    E   has no effect on the rate of production of the fluid.

VIII.14 Sodium reabsorption in the nephron is:

    A   greater in the distal than in the proximal convoluted tubule
    B   only achieved in exchange for potassium excretion
    C   the major energy consuming activity of the kidney
    D   the main object of the countercurrent multiplier system
    E   dependent on the glomerular filtration rate as well as aldosterone.

VIII.15 The carotid body chemoreceptors:

    A   are stimulated by a fall of arterial O_2 tension
    B   are inhibited by a fall of arterial pH
    C   produce reflex peripheral vasoconstriction
    D   are responsible for increased ventilation in a patient with carbon monoxide poisoning
    E   have a very high tissue blood flow.

VIII.16 Which of the following are used in the calculation of oxygen availability:

A   cardiac output
B   the oxygen equivalent of haemoglobin
C   physiological shunt
D   the dead-space ratio
E   oxygen saturation.

VIII.17 In the normal pulmonary vascular bed:

A   the mean pulmonary arterial pressure is a constant fraction of the mean aortic pressure
B   the pulmonary vascular resistance is lower than the systemic vascular resistance
C   there is approximately 50% of the blood volume
D   the "wedge" pressure equals pulmonary capillary pressure
E   hypoxia causes reflex vasodilation.

VIII.18 Surfactant:

A   reduces surface tension within the lung
B   consists of ribosomes and nucleotides
C   is an insoluble lipoprotein layer
D   is a sulphonated hydrocarbon
E   will only reduce alveolar surface tension in alveoli of radius greater than 6 microns.

VIII.19 The oxyhaemoglobin dissociation curve for human haemoglobin A:

A   is independent of barometric pressure
B   yields more oxygen to the tissues when shifted to the left
C   can be unaffected by metabolic acidosis because the acidosis reduces red cell 2,3-DPG
D   has a p50 of 26.6 mm Hg
E   shifts to the left with hypothermia.

VIII.20 The factors which prevent changes in intrapleural pressure being directly proportional to volume changes in the lung are:

A   that the lungs contain smooth muscle
B   that surface tension in alveoli gives rise to excess elasticity
C   lung compliance
D   that elasticity is reduced but not abolished by surfactant
E   that intrapleural pressure varies with different phases of the respiratory cycle.

VIII.21 The following will block alpha-adrenergic receptors:

- **A** trimetaphan
- **B** phenoxybenzamine
- **C** indoramin
- **D** phentolamine
- **E** chlorpromazine.

VIII.22 Beta adrenergic blockade is produced by:

- **A** labetalol
- **B** metaraminol
- **C** verapamil
- **D** oxprenalol
- **E** disopyramide.

VIII.23 The following drugs will lower the mean blood pressure if injected intravenously:

- **A** phentolamine
- **B** isoprenaline
- **C** 10% calcium chloride
- **D** thiopentone
- **E** metaraminol.

VIII.24 An increase in cardiac output follows treatment with:

- **A** reserpine
- **B** alpha-methyldopa
- **C** hydralazine
- **D** oxprenolol
- **E** guanethidine.

VIII.25 Proteinase inhibitors suitable for antagonising fibrinolysis include:

- **A** streptokinase
- **B** tranexamic acid
- **C** stanozolol
- **D** aprotinin
- **E** epsilon amino caproic acid.

VIII.26 Frusemide:

A   acts only on the distal convoluted tubule
B   must not be given with cephalosporins
C   the diuresis is complete by 6 hours
D   causes hyperglycaemia
E   potassium supplements should always be given.

VIII.27 When dextran solutions are used as blood substitutes:

A   they may interfere with subsequent cross-matching
B   the intravascular volume increases by more than the volume infused
C   they must be infused in a fast running centrally placed intravenous line
D   rapid infusion will lower the plasma calcium
E   dextran 40 has been associated with renal damage.

VIII.28 The sulphonylureas:

A   have a half-life in man of 18 hours
B   act mainly by enhancing insulin action
C   are ideal in the grossly obese
D   are safe in chronic renal failure
E   can be used as a diagnostic test in the incipient diabetic.

VIII.29 Trichloroethylene:

A   is an isomer of trichloroethane
B   has a high fat solubility
C   is a good analgesic in sub-anaesthetic concentrations
D   was coloured blue originally to distinguish it from chloroform
E   cannot be used in temperature-compensated vaporisers.

VIII.30 Nitrous oxide:

A   is less soluble than oxygen
B   only 1.2% is metabolised, the remainder is eliminated unchanged
C   has a MAC of 105%
D   may cause megaloblastic anaemia
E   impurities include ammonia.

VIII.31 Cyclopropane:

　　A　does not depress hepatic function
　　B　is associated with postoperative nausea and vomiting
　　C　may induce postoperative shock, particularly after hypercapnoea
　　D　interferes with normal blood coagulation
　　E　is contraindicated in children.

VIII.32 In the metabolism of these drugs:

　　A　morphine forms a conjugated glucuronide
　　B　penicillin is mainly hydrolysed
　　C　one of the major metabolic product of halothane is monofluoroacetic acid
　　D　pethidine metabolism requires catechol-o-methyltransferase
　　E　cocaine is hydrolysed.

VIII.33 The following statements are true:

　　A　noradrenaline is a pure alpha adrenergic receptor stimulant
　　B　tetracycline is absorbed better if taken before meals
　　C　atropine prevents bronchoconstriction caused by cigarette smoking
　　D　penicillin was the first antibiotic to be used clinically
　　E　the atropinising dose in a healthy man is 0.04 mg/kg.

VIII.34 Aminoplex 12:

　　A　has an osmolarity of 350 mosmol/litre
　　B　contains 15 G nitrogen/litre
　　C　contains 35 mmol sodium/litre
　　D　contains no carbohydrate source
　　E　contains 30 mmol potassium/litre.

VIII.35 Prilocaine:

　　A　is excreted in the urine
　　B　0.5% solution is suitable for intravenous (Bier's) block
　　C　methaemoglobinaemia is common but usually clinically unimportant
　　D　is less toxic than lignocaine
　　E　may produce sleepiness.

VIII.36 The following potentiate the effect of non-depolarising neuromuscular blocking agents:

- A   hypokalaemia
- B   hypothermia
- C   hypercalcaemia
- D   hypomagnesaemia
- E   cephazolin.

VIII.37 Ecothiopate is used in the treatment of:

- A   glaucoma
- B   myaesthenia gravis
- C   hyperhidrosis
- D   phenothiazine induced sedation
- E   depression.

VIII.38 Aspirin:

- A   can cause iron deficiency anaemia
- B   is secreted in breast milk
- C   is an antipyretic
- D   has analeptic properties
- E   causes tinnitus in large doses.

VIII.39 Histamine release follows clinical dosage of:

- A   pentagastrin
- B   ranitidine
- C   alcuronium
- D   etomidate
- E   suxamethonium.

VIII.40 Convulsions are produced by:

- A   diphenhydramine
- B   penicillin
- C   phenobarbitone
- D   enflurane
- E   acetazolamide.

VIII.41 Blood volume measurement:

  A requires measurement of red cell volume which can satisfactorily be obtained from haemoglobin estimation.

  B may be estimated by dilution of radioactive albumin.

  C requires simultaneous measurement of radioactive sodium dilution and labelled red cell dilution.

  D blood loss can be estimated fairly accurately by haemoglobin dilution in swab washings

  E blood loss may be measured in acute haemorrhage by reduction in haemoglobin concentration.

VIII.42 Oxygen content measurement:

  A may be made directly using a fuel cell

  B necessitates haemolysis of the blood sample prior to estimation

  C is affected by carbon monoxide in cigarette smoke

  D in the van Slyke apparatus, oxygen is absorbed by acid pyrogallol

  E by the van Slyke method requires haemolysis of the blood sample.

VIII.43 A liquid will boil:

  A when the saturated vapour pressure equals atmospheric pressure

  B at a higher temperature if the ambient pressure is reduced

  C at a temperature above its critical temperature

  D as its critical pressure is reduced

  E when the molecular energy is so great that all molecules transfer to the gas phase.

VIII.44 The following would be normal pressures in a fit adult:

  A aortic root 120/0 mm Hg

  B radial artery 130/75 mm Hg

  C right ventricle 25/8 mm Hg

  D end capillary 17 mm Hg (mean)

  E right atrium 2 cm H_2O (mean).

VIII.45 For a variable that shows a normal distribution:

  A the modal, median and mean values will be the same

  B the variance will equal the standard deviation

  C as the sample size increases, the sample mean will be a better estimate of the population mean

  D the coefficient of variation is a constant

  E a value more than 2 standard deviations from the mean is abnormal.

VIII.46 During induction of anaesthesia with a volatile agent:

A a few deep breaths at the start of induction will ensure the alveolar concentration will equal the inspired concentration

B the arterial and venous blood concentrations will be the same

C "overpressure" is possible only with the more volatile agents

D right-to-left shunts will speed induction

E left-to-right shunts will speed induction.

VIII.47 4PH = 7 35, PaO_2 = 16.2 kPa (122 mm Hg), $PaCO_2$ = 3.5 kPa (26 mm Hg) is compatible with:

A a base excess of −10 mmol/L

B FIO_2 = 0.24

C a bicarbonate of 6 mmol/L

D a partially compensated respiratory alkalosis

E an overcompensated metabolic alkalosis.

VIII.48 Glomerular filtration rate:

A is approximately 125 ml/min

B is influenced by the intrinsic pressure within Bowman's capsule

C measurement must involve a substance which is not reabsorbed or secreted into the tubule

D is reduced in ureteric obstruction

E the normal filtration fraction is approximately 0.2.

VIII.49 The following help prevent electrical injury to the patient in the operating theatre:

A an internal pacemaker

B a common earth point

C an isolating transformer

D non-polarising electrodes

E diathermy at ground potential.

VIII.50 In the Severinghaus electrode:

A the electrode makes contact with sodium bicarbonate solution

B the electrode is made of CO_2-sensitive glass

C Teflon may be used as a filter to prevent the passage of H^+ ions

D the electrode works independently of temperature

E requires frequent calibration.

VIII.51 Humidification:

A hot water humidifiers normally operate at 60°C to pasteurise the water in the humidifier
B gas-driven nebulisers utilise the Bernoulli effect
C ultrasonic nebulisers may produce fluid overload
D nebulised water particles less than 5 microns in diameter pass directly into the alveoli on inspiration
E the normal level of humidity at 37°C in the upper trachea is approximately 20 G per cubic metre.   35 gm/m³

VIII.52 Transducers:

A are devices which change one form of energy into another
B in a strain gauge, resistance increases as the wire is stretched
C in capacitance transducers, the capacitor is mounted within the body of the transducer
D the transducer diaphragm should be zeroed at the level of the right atrium
E transducer calibration should always be carried out with the dome vertical to ensure removal of air.

VIII.53 Turbulent flow:

A is proportional to the square of the pressure
B is proportional to the length of the tube
C will become laminar if the radius of the tube is reduced
D is independent of the viscosity of the fluid
E is independent of the density of the fluid.

VIII.54 Saturated vapour pressure:

A is dependent on the ambient pressure
B increases linearly with ambient temperature
C is the pressure exerted at equilibrium by a vapour in contact with its liquid
D of water at body temperature exceeds the normal $PaCO_2$
E can be estimated from the molecular weight by using Henry's law.

VIII.55 Vaporisers:

A the "copper kettle" supplies a saturated vapour
B with vaporisers in series, the liquid with the lower boiling point should be vaporised first
C IPPV can result in concentrations of vapour higher than that set on the dial when the vaporiser is outside the circuit
D at 2 atmospheres and at a given dial setting the concentration of a vapour will be halved but the tension remains the same
E the Goldman vaporiser produces up to 5 per cent v/v of halothane.

VIII.56 The following are true:

A   the application of logarithms can be used to simplify all arithmetic manipulations

B   a logarithmic function is a power function

C   a graphical representation of $y = ax + c$ would be a straight line

D   a hyperbolic function is one that is asymptotic to the axes

E   if the product of two variables is a constant then the relation is hyperbolic.

VIII.57 Gas volumes can be accurately measured by:

A   Wright respirometer

B   Benedict-Roth wet spirometer

C   Vitalograph

D   pneumotachograph

E   dry gas meter.

VIII.58 Viscosity:

A   may affect the velocity of established turbulent flow

B   of blood varies in direct proportion to the plasma protein concentrations

C   increased viscosity uniformly reduces blood flow

D   low temperature raises blood viscosity

E   helium improves gas flow through an orifice by reducing viscosity.

VIII.59 Heat loss:

A   the amount of heat lost by sweating may increase tenfold under certain conditions

B   convection is an unimportant route of heat loss from the body

C   the human body acts as an almost perfect radiator, making heat loss due to radiation a significant factor

D   the normal surface temperature of the human body is 32–35°C

E   the normal core temperature of the human body varies diurnally by 0. 4°C.

VIII.60 In the measurement of flow:

A   the cardiac output is indirectly proportional to the area under the dye dilution curve

B   changes in the ratio of reduced haemoglobin to oxyhaemoglobin will affect cardiac output measurements with indocyanine green

C   blood flow = oxygen consumption divided by the arteriovenous difference in oxygen content

D   glomerular filtration is measured using I^{131} hippuran

E   Doppler ultrasonic flowmeters use frequencies up to 10 MHertz.

Paper VIII Answers

VIII.1 FTTTF

A & E are true, but are nicotinic actions.

VIII.2 FTFFT

A On the contrary, it supplies the energy for contraction.

B AMP is not a high energy phosphate compound.

C Energy is stored as ATP along the chain, but is not an integral part of the system.

D However, anaerobic catabolism of glucose produces fewer ATP molecules per molecule of glucose.

VIII.3 FTTTF

Starling's law is **C**. **B** and **D** are re-statements of it that require assumptions about the relation of end-diastolic muscle fibre length to pressure and volume. **A** and **B** may or may not be true but are not consequent on the law. Remember that the law can be readily demonstrated in vitro but in intact animals and man autonomic and other effects usually override it.

VIII.4 TTTFT

The Valsalva manoeuvre is a forced expiration against a closed glottis. A full understanding of it is essential to the understanding of cardiovascular homeostasis and an account will be found in any good textbook of physiology.

D The blood pressure does not remain raised. The peripheral resistance does rise and that is why an overshoot of blood pressure occurs at the end of the manoeuvre.

VIII.5 FFFFT

A The barrier exists at every capillary.

B It is more permeable in the neonate.

C,E All drugs cross the barrier to some extent although the time to equilibration will be very prolonged compared to transfer across other capillaries.

D Little catecholamine will transfer from the systemic circulation, but they are synthesised within the CNS.

VIII.6 TTTTT

It is helpful to be familiar with a "circuit diagram" of the proposed mechanism of the gate theory and the transmission and reception of nociceptive stimuli.

VIII.7 FTTTF

Prostaglandins are a family of compounds found in a wide variety of tissues and having a wide variety of biological actions. Chemically they are fatty acids and many have now been synthesised.

VIII.8 TFTTT

B   The amount of endogenous vasopressin in the circulation of normal individuals is too small to affect blood pressure.

C   It is frequently given as snuff, absorbed from the nasal mucosa.

VIII.9 FTTFT

A   The atomic weight of sodium (23) is less than potassium (39) and so one might expect sodium to be (in general) more readily diffusible. However the hydrated sodium ion is larger than the hydrated potassium ion.

D   Its use as an osmotic diuretic depends on its not crossing membranes.

VIII.10 FFTTT

A   It is initiated by sodium influx.

B   Velocity is constant along a fibre of a given diameter.

C   In other words, the action potential "leaps" from node to node.

D   There are large pain fibres (A delta); there are no large temperature fibres.

VIII.11 TTTFT

D   Streptokinase is not produced in man but by a bacterium.
Urokinase is of human origin.

VIII.12 TFTFT

B   Not necessarily.
D   Anaphylatoxins are C3a and C5a.

VIII.13 FTFTT

A   The figure is correct, but the units should be mm of water.
D   This test is jugular compression.

VIII.14 FFTFT

A   The distal tubule exerts fine control, but the majority is
absorbed in the proximal convoluted tubule.
B   Can equally be exchanged for other cations eg H^+.
D   No – this is concerned primarily with the setting up of a
hypertonic medulla to increase the reabsorption of water,
although sodium reabsorption is the way in which this is
done.

VIII.15 TFTFT

B   Fall of pH = acidaemia = stimulation of the
chemoreceptors.
C   This is a reflex caused by stimulation of the
chemoreceptors by whatever stimulus not by hypoxia
per se.
D,E   The blood flow is so high that the oxygen requirements
can be supplied by the dissolved oxygen.

VIII.16 TTFFT

"Available oxygen" is a concept for which the cardiac output is multiplied by the total oxygen in the blood, combined and dissolved. Shunt and dead space will reduce the availability of oxygen by affecting the saturation but an actual measure of them is not needed for the calculation.

VIII.17 FTFFF

A,B, The pressure in a system is the product of the cardiac output and the resistance. The resistances change independently so **A** must be false, and the pulmonary arterial pressure is low for the same flow so **B** must be true.
C   One litre, increasing by about 400 ml on lying down.
D   In normal subjects, the "wedge" pressure equals the left atrial pressure.
E   Hypoxia causes vasoconstriction, mainly by a local response.

VIII.18 TFTFF

B,C,D Bad question because these are mutually exclusive.
E   It will affect surface tension whatever the alveolar radius.

VIII.19 TFTTT

B   The leftward shift maintains haemoglobin saturation at a lower PaO_2, thereby reducing oxygen availability at the tissues.

VIII.20 FTTTT

A   True, in the bronchi and blood vessels, but this doesn't prevent intrapleural pressure changes being directly proportional to changes in lung volume.

VIII.21 FTTTT

A Trimetaphan is a ganglion blocking agent. = *arene Nii*.
B A long-term alpha-blocker used, eg, in phaeochromocytoma.
C Used in the treatment of hypertension.
D Take care: it is easy to misread phentolamine (alpha-blocker) for pentolinium (ganglion blocker).

VIII.22 TFFTF

B Alpha agonist, peripheral vasoconstriction.
C Calcium antagonist.
E An anti-arrhythmic with no action at beta-receptors, although it is a negative inotrope.

VIII.23 TTFTF

In a question which gives a list of drugs, it is likely that the drugs will be contrasting ones. Take care to answer correctly – the important word here is "lower" the blood pressure; it could just as easily have said "raise' and then the opposite answers would be true.

A A ganglion blocker.
B Pure beta effects: beta1 – cardiac output will increase, but beta2 vasodilatation will balance this; mean blood pressure will be little altered or will fall, diastolic pressure will fall.
E A sympathomimetic amine with both alpha and beta effects.

VIII.24 FFTFF

A,B No significant change.
C Central sympathetic action.
D Reduced due to impairment of the haemodynamic response to adrenaline.
E Venous pooling leads to decreased venous return.

VIII.25 FTFTT

A Streptokinase is a plasminogen activator.
C Stanozolol is a testosterone derivative and activates plasminogen.
D Trasylol – more usually associated with pancreatitis where it is used to antagonise pancreatic enzymes.

VIII.26 FFTTF

A   The most important site of action is in the ascending loop of Henle; it also acts on the PCT.

B   Care was needed with the first generation drugs such as cephaloridine. The third-generation cephalosporins and cephamycins do not have this problem.

C   Diuresis will be complete sooner if given intravenously.

D   Large doses may reveal latent diabetes or increase insulin requirements.

E   Not if the serum potassium is high, for instance in renal failure.

VIII.27 TTFFF

C   This applies to irritant (eg amino-acids) or very hypertonic (eg 50% dextrose) solutions; it does not apply to dextrans.

D   There is confusion here with the citrate in blood or plasma infusions.

E   The high molecular weight dextrans, eg dextran 110, have been connected with renal damage.

VIII.28 FFFFF

A   The half-life depends on the particular drug.

B   They increase secretion, unlike the biguanides, and needs about 30% normal beta cell function.

C   Best avoided in the obese unless dieting and weight loss has not helped.

D   Must be used with caution, especially chlorpropamide because it is not metabolised. Some of the metabolites are also hypoglycaemic.

E   No, but tolbutamide is sometimes used in the diagnosis of insulinoma.

VIII.29 FTTTF

A   Basic organic chemistry. Ethylene is $H_2C=CH_2$; ethane is H_3C-CH_3.

E   Though often given from a Boyle's bottle, there are vaporisers available, eg the Tritec.

VIII.30 FFTTF

A   It is 15 times more soluble

B   Nitrous oxide is eliminated entirely unchanged.

C   A theoretical figure (at 1 atmosphere) calculable because MAC's are additive.

E   NO and NO_2.

VIII.31 TTTFF

D   No effect on coagulation – anaesthetics generally do not have a significant effect.

E   No – often used for paediatric gaseous induction, though less now.

VIII.32 TFFFT

A   The major pathway for morphine.

B   Penicillin is excreted mainly via the kidneys.

C   There are a number of products, including trifluoroacetic acid. Cl^- and Br^- are more easily removed from the halothane molecule than is F^-.

D   The interaction here is with mono-amine oxidase inhibitors which slow the metabolism of pethidine and can also cause a hyperpyrexic reaction. Pethidine is hydrolysed, partially conjugated, and also demethylated.

VIII.33 FTTTT

A   Mild beta effect too.

B   Difficult one, tetracycline absorption depends upon local gastric pH but there is also the complication that tetracyclines can be chelated by food, eg, the calcium in milk.

D   Sulphanilamide was used before penicillin but, not being a compound obtained from a living organism, it is not strictly an antibiotic although it is an antimicrobial drug.

VIII.34 FFTTT

A   Much more hypertonic – 840 mOsmol/litre.

B   Contains 12 grams of nitrogen – hence the name.

VIII.35 FTTTT

A   It is metabolised in the liver, like lignocaine, and little reaches the urine.

B   Recent observations suggest that it is better, because less toxic, than bupivacaine.

D   "Less toxic" implies at an equipotent dose, ie a reflection of the therapeutic ratio. On a comparative basis, if procaine is given a safety factor of 1, bupivacaine is 1.7, lignocaine is 2 and prilocaine is the safest at 3

VIII.36 TTFFF

A   An increase in the [K]i:[K]o ratio increases both the resting potential and transmitter release (conflicting actions). The actual clinical effect is variable.

B A   complex matter: hypothermia affects many aspects, physiological and pharamacological, of neuromuscular transmission.

C,D   A raised concentration of magnesium or a lowered concentration of calcium can potentiate the non-depolarising drugs.

E   Some antibiotics potentiate, especially aminoglycosides and polymyxins.

VIII.37 TFFFF

B,C,D,E   Ecothiopate is an anticholinesterase which does not cross the blood-brain barrier and is only used locally in the treatment of glaucoma because of its prolonged effect which lasts 4 to 6 weeks.

VIII.38 TTTFT

A   Erosions leading to gastric bleeding.

C   Especially in children.

D   It is a metabolic stimulant and stimulates respiration secondary to this, but is not a direct analeptic.

VIII.39 FFFFT

Generally, a very awkward question. There are very few drugs which have not, at some time, been shown to cause histamine release. What really matters is if the release is clinically important. Contrast the wording of VI.40

A   Pentagastrin mimics histamine but it does not cause release.

B   Ranitidine is an H2-antagonist. That does not mean it is incapable of causing systemic release of histamine but it has not been described.

C   Alcuronium will cause release only in excessive dosage.

E   Release by suxamethonium is less than by tubocurarine.

VIII.40 TTFTF

A   Antihistamines commonly produce drowsiness in overdose but can cause convulsions, especially in children.

B   Not a feature of systemic toxicity but may follow intrathecal administration.

C   Anticonvulsant.

E   Carbonic anhydrase inhibitor.

VIII.41 FFFTF

- **A** Requires labelled red blood cells, haemoglobin concentration may vary for many reasons.
- **B** Measuring albumin can only measure plasma volume.
- **C** Radioactive sodium measures the total extracellular fluid volume.
- **E** Measurement of the packed cell volume is often used in the acute situation but neither gives an accurate value.

VIII.42 TTFFT

- **A** True – lex-O_2-con.
- **C** The method of measurement is unaffected although the actual oxygen content will be reduced.
- **D** Alkaline pyrogallol.

VIII.43 TFFFF

- **B** Boiling point is reduced if there is a reduction in ambient pressure.
- **C** Critical temperature is that temperature above which a substance cannot be liquified, despite alterations in pressure.
- **D** Critical pressure is a property of the substance and cannot be changed.
- **E** The liquid would explode!

VIII.44 FTFTT

- **A** This is the LV pressure. Aortic root is 120/80.
- **C** The opposite of **A**: RV is 25/0.

VIII.45 TFTFF

- **B** The standard deviation is the square root of the variance.
- **D** The CV is the mean divided by the standard deviation and will depend on the shape of the distribution, ie how peaked it is.
- **E** By definition, 5% of normal values lie outside this range.

VIII.46 FFFFT

Poor marks here must be rectified by reading and understanding.

A,B Only at equilibrium, and that is not practically attainable even with nitrous oxide.

C Overpressure is possible with all agents except nitrous oxide.

D,E An extremely complex subject, further complicated by how the shunt will change as cardiac output changes with the induction of anaesthesia. However, other things being equal, a right-to-left shunt will dilute the anaesthetic agent, and a left-to-right shunt will increase the concentration.

VIII.47 TTFFF

It is a metabolic acidosis with respiratory compensation. The patient must be having oxygen therapy.

B The maximum PaO_2 with an FiO_2 of 0.24 is about 135 mm Hg assuming a normal atmospheric pressure and $PACO_2$.

C The bicarbonate would be 18 mmol/l.

D,E The pH for either condition would have to be above 7.4.

VIII.48 TTTTT

D Back pressure effects.

VIII.49 TTTFF

A Rather than an external pacemaker.

B For all electrical equipment attached to the patient.

D Improves signal quality, no effect on safety.

E This is meaningless, though the output circuit should be isolated from earth.

VIII.50 TFFFT

You should be able to draw the CO_2 electrode with its constituent parts.

B It is a modified pH electrode – sensitive to H^+.

C The membrane, which may be made of Teflon, is permeable to CO_2 but not to liquids or solids.

D Temperature must be controlled to 37 +/− 0.1°C.

VIII.51 FTTFF

  A   Normally 40–45°C, occasionally 60.
  D   A diameter of 1 micron is the ideal size to pass into the alveoli.
  E   35G per cubic metre.

VIII.52 TTTTF

  A   They are not simply for measurement of blood pressure
  E   The vertical position is correct to exclude air, but it should be calibrated in the position in which it is to be used.

VIII.53 FFFTF

  You must know the formulae relating flow to pressure and the answers to this question follow from them.
  C   Reducing the radius will increase velocity and flow will be more likely to be turbulent. If the same flow is directed into many smaller tubes in parallel then the velocity will be unaffected and flow will remain laminar (eg the pneumotachograph head).

VIII.54 FFTTF

  A   A basic principle that you must understand is that SVP depends ONLY on the temperature and the nature of the liquid.
  B   It is an approximately exponential relation that is different for each liquid.
  D   SVP of water at 37°C = 6.3 kPa (47 mm Hg).
  E   There is no way of estimating SVP from molecular weight, and Henry's law concerns solubility of gas in a liquid.

VIII.55 TTTTF

  A   This can then be diluted by fresh gas to give the required concentration.
  B   The more volatile liquid is less likely to condense in (and contaminate) the less volatile liquid.
  C   This can happen if back-pressure causes fresh gas already loaded with agent to re-enter the chamber; modern designs eliminate this. IPPV can always give high concentrations if the vaporiser is inside the circuit.
  D   1% of 1 atmosphere = 1/2% of 2 atmospheres. Remember that the SVP is unchanged.
  E   At 8 L/min, at "ON", the Goldman will deliver 3% halothane.

VIII.56 FTTFT

Mathematics can be quite important because it can be used to describe so many principles in the basic anaesthetic sciences. If you find mathematical manipulation difficult try at least to understand what it means in simple English and perhaps an illustration from physiology or pharmacology.

A,B Only to multiplication or division, by adding or subtracting powers.

D,E eg the so-called metabolic hyperbola (CO_2 output = VA × $PaCO_2$) that results when alveolar ventilation is changed and the resulting $PaCO_2$ measured. This is asymptotic to the axes, but it is not necessarily so; there may be other constants, eg k = (a-m) × (b-n) where m and n define the asymptotes.

VIII.57 FTTTT

A The Wright's respirometer is inaccurate for continuous flow or at high or low flow rates.

D True, provided the flow signal is integrated with respect to time, eg in the Servo ventilator.

VIII.58 FTFTF

A Density only, except at the onset of turbulent flow when Reynold's number is important – note that here it says ESTABLISHED turbulent flow.

C No – the reduction varies with vessel diameter and is more marked near the vessel wall where flow is low anyway.

E Flow is density dependent through an orifice.

VIII.59 TFTTT

B Convection is important, by warming air adjacent to the body and setting up convection currents

VIII.60 TFTFT

A A lower output = less dilution of the dye = a larger area under the curve.

B Indocyanine green is used because changes in oxygenation do not alter the spectrophotometry (read about "isobestic point"). Note that this is not a question about oxygenation affecting cardiac output.

C This is the basic principle of indicator dilution techniques (Fick).

D Hippuran is used to measure renal blood flow.

IX.1 The autonomic nervous system:

A is part of the peripheral nervous system, but independant of conscious control

B is the efferent pathway to all viscera

C comprises all the efferent fibres in the body except those to voluntary muscle

D transmits visceral sensation

E the main parasympathetic outflow is from the cranial and sacral regions.

IX.2 Iron absorption:

A is usually about 15 mg per day

B is regulated by body stores

C takes place in the terminal ileum

D is stored in the intestinal cells in combination with apoferritin

E is increased by a high phosphate concentration in the diet.

IX.3 The venous return:

A will be increased by a deep inspiration

B is increased initially on assuming upright posture

C is not affected by arteriovenous fistulae

D falls in moderate exercise

E is regulated directly by aldosterone.

IX.4 In the foetal circulation:

A blood in the ductus arteriosus is more saturated than blood in the ductus venosus

B blood can pass from the IVC to the aorta without passing through the heart

C blood in the umbilical veins is 50% saturated

D the PO_2 in the umbilical artery is 2.7 kPa (20 mm Hg)

E blood passing to the brain and arms is better oxygenated than that passing to the lower parts of the body.

IX.5 Nerve conduction:

A the conduction velocity of the fastest motor fibres in man is 50 metres/sec

B the resting membrane potential in human motor nerves is caused by constant leakage of ions

C sympathetic nerves are always unmyelinated

D conduction velocity is dependent upon local oxygenation

E is independent of serum magnesium concentrations.

IX.6 Unilateral damage to the cerebellum in man produces:
A disturbances of posture
B disturbances of voluntary movement
C intellectual impairment, particularly if connections to the dominant hemisphere are involved
D incoordinated movement, made worse by closing the eyes
E ipsilateral loss of position sense.

IX.7 Aldosterone:
A is formed in the zona reticularis of the adrenal gland
B has a half life of 24 hours
C acts on the distal convoluted tubule of the kidney
D increases the level of Angiotensin II in the blood
E is released in response to a high intake of potassium in the diet.

IX.8 The thyroid hormones:
A are synthesised from alanine
B are active in the L-form
C are highly bound to plasma proteins
D are partly bound to albumin
E their calorigenic actions are "governed" by the corticosteroids.

IX.9 Intraocular pressure:
A is directly proportional to the blood pressure
B is increased by coughing
C is reduced by hyperventilation
D depends on the angle of the anterior chamber
E is decreased by osmotic diuretics.

IX.10 The following gastric secretions are essential to life:
A HCl
B intrinsic factor
C pepsin
D rennin
E gastrin.

IX.11 Factors known to enhance fibrinolysis include:
- **A** menstruation
- **B** exercise
- **C** hypercapnoea
- **D** venous stasis and occlusion
- **E** incompatible blood transfusion.

IX.12 Factors which predispose to the development of a hypersensitivity reaction to an intravenous anaesthetic induction agent include:
- **A** atopy
- **B** pregnancy
- **C** previous exposure to the agent
- **D** stress
- **E** preoperative hypovolaemia.

IX.13 Cerebrospinal fluid:
- **A** the specific gravity of 1003–1009 depends little on the protein content
- **B** pH is alkaline relative to serum
- **C** total volume is about 135 ml of which 25% is in the spinal space
- **D** contains no antibodies
- **E** contains up to 5 lymphocytes per cu mm.

IX.14 Mildly impaired glomerular function produces abnormal values of:
- **A** plasma bicarbonate
- **B** blood urea
- **C** serum phosphate
- **D** creatinine clearance
- **E** serum magnesium.

IX.15 The central chemoreceptors:
- **A** are more sensitive to changes in the composition of CSF than of blood
- **B** are uninfluenced by changes in arterial oxygen content
- **C** are pH dependent
- **D** are sensitive to local CSF bicarbonate changes
- **E** are probably not bathed directly by CSF.

IX.16 For a group of alveoli that are under ventilated but which have normal perfusion:

    A   the PaO_2 will fall

    B   the $PaCO_2$ will fall

    C   the V/Q ratio will fall

    D   the pulmonary artery saturation will be low

    E   the contribution from well ventilated alveoli will bring the overall $PaCO_2$ to normal but not the PaO_2.

IX.17 The normal pulmonary circulation:

    A   in the foetus, only 15% of the cardiac output goes to the lungs

    B   during passage, angiotensin II is inactivated

    C   PGF2-alpha causes vasoconstriction

    D   the velocity of blood in the root of the pulmonary artery is the same as that in the aorta

    E   capillary pressure is about 10 mm Hg.

IX.18 Alveolar minute ventilation:

    A   is equal to total minute ventilation minus the dead space

    B   can be calculated from the alveolar air equation

    C   is equal to (tidal volume minus dead space) multiplied by respiratory rate

    D   is approximately 8 ml/kg per breath at rest

    E   varies with posture.

IX.19 The oxyhaemoglobin dissociation curve is:

    A   a curve relating quantity of oxygen combining with haemoglobin to the partial pressure of oxygen in the gas with which the blood is equilibrated

    B   the dissociation constant of oxygen

    C   a reflection of the efficiency of oxygen transport

    D   the same shape and position for haemoglobin A and myoglobin

    E   only sigmoid shaped in vivo.

IX.20 In acute hepatic failure:

    A   the prothrombin time is prolonged

    B   serum alkaline phosphatase can be normal

    C   serum albumin may be below 10 gm/L

    D   bromsulphthalein excretion test is only valid in the absence of jaundice

    E   serum LDH is a sensitive index of hepatocellular damage.

IX.21 The Rauwolfia alkaloids:

A   have been used to treat schizophrenia
B   may interact with inotropic agents given intravenously
C   are incompatible with beta-adrenergic blocking drugs
D   cause psychological depression
E   deplete the tissue stores of noradrenaline.

IX.22 Alpha adrenergic blockade is produced by:

A   phentolamine
B   isoprenaline
C   labetalol
D   indoramin
E   phenylephrine.

IX.23 Thiazide diuretics lower blood pressure in the hypertensive patient by:

A   a mild negative inotropism
B   a reduction in blood volume
C   a reduction in vascular tone
D   a central depressant action
E   reducing catecholamine re-uptake.

IX.24 Digitalis:

A   increases the contractile force of the normal human heart
B   dilates arteriolar and venous beds in the forearms of normal subjects
C   produces a rise in serum potassium
D   impairs electrical defibrillation of the heart
E   hypothyroidism augments the inotropic and arrhythmogenic properties of digitalis.

IX.25 Pharmacological methods of deep venous thrombosis prevention include:

A   subcutaneous sodium heparin
B   aspirin
C   stanozolol
D   Ancrod
E   streptokinase.

IX.26 The benzothiazide diuretics:

- A   cause potassium loss
- B   cause relative loss of bicarbonate
- C   block exchange of sodium for hydrogen
- D   have a direct effect on peripheral vascular resistance
- E   cause sodium loss.

IX.27 The following drugs can be reversed by naloxone:

- A   thiopentone
- B   methadone
- C   glutethimide
- D   pethidine
- E   diamorphine.

IX.28 Metformin:

- A   does not cause the lactic acidosis sometimes seen with phenformin
- B   does not cause hypoglycaemia in normal subjects
- C   should not be used with a sulphonylurea
- D   does not work unless there are some functioning islet cells
- E   is contra-indicated in the alcoholic patient.

IX.29 Thiopentone is a short lasting barbiturate because:

- A   it is metabolised by the liver
- B   it is redistributed to muscle
- C   it is specifically bound to the reticular activating system
- D   it is given by rapid intravenous injection
- E   it induces tachyphylaxis.

IX.30 Theories of anaesthesia:

- A   the potency of volatile anaesthetics is related to their lipid solubility
- B   the pressure reversal theory is only applicable to volatile anaesthetics
- C   M.A.C. correlates best with lipid solubility
- D   the narcotic potential of inert gases and vapours is inversely proportional to their vapour pressure
- E   the theory of narcosis which postulated that anaesthesia was related to the formation of hydrate microcrystals was suggested by Pauling.

IX.31 Ether:

    A has a boiling point of 35° C

    B has a saturated vapour pressure of 350 at 20° C

    C induces a tachycardia by vagal depression

    D is contraindicated if adrenaline is to be infiltrated

    E does not cross the placental barrier.

IX.32 In the excretion of these drugs:

    A phenobarbitone is excreted mainly in the bile

    B ether is excreted partly through the skin

    C at least 60–80% of halothane is excreted through the lungs

    D neostigmine is excreted unchanged

    E fazadinium is excreted mainly via the liver.

IX.33 Effects of chlorpromazine include:

    A antipruritic action

    B anticholinergic action

    C bradycardia

    D potentiation of neuromuscular blocking agents during anaesthesia

    E constipation.

IX.34 Tinnitus is a side-effect of:

    A codeine

    B aspirin

    C cocaine

    D nikethamide

    E amphetamine.

IX.35 Intravenous lignocaine :

    A depresses pharyngeal reflexes

    B depresses respiration

    C depresses laryngeal reflexes

    D produces convulsions

    E relieves laryngeal spasm.

IX.36 Suxamethonium:

A   increases intra-ocular pressure
B   decomposes in solution if not stored at 4°C
C   should not be used in patients who have sustained severe burns
D   raises the serum potassium
E   pains are more likely in ambulant patients.

IX.37 Atracurium:

A   is a medium acting neuromuscular blocking drug
B   is frequently associated with histamine release
C   is metabolised by Hoffman elimination
D   is contraindicated in patients with renal disease
E   is more cardiovascularly depressant than d-tubocurarine.

IX.38 Dependance occurs in patients treated with:

A   methadone
B   phenoperidine
C   buprenorphine
D   nalorphine
E   pentazocine.

IX.39 The following drugs have been implicated in causing venous thrombosis:

A   methohexitone
B   pancuronium
C   thiopentone ✓
D   propanidid ✓
E   hydroxydione.

IX.40 The following affect sympathetic responses in man:

A   guanethidine
B   sodium nitroprusside
C   tricyclic antidepressants
D   diazoxide
E   promethazine.

IX.41 The pneumotachograph:

- A directly measures pressure change across a resistance
- B the resistance must have a configuration that ensures laminar gas flow
- C is not suitable for accurate breath-by-breath monitoring
- D accuracy is affected by temperature change
- E accuracy is unaffected by alterations in gas composition.

IX.42 Oxygen concentration measurement:

- A oxygen is a paramagnetic gas because the molecule has unpaired electrons in the outer shell
- B in a paramagnetic analyser the two glass spheres are filled with oxygen
- C in a paramagnetic analyser, rotation of the dumb-bell is balanced by tension in a suspending filament
- D in a null-deflection analyser, an opposing magnetic field prevents movement of the dumb-bell
- E water vapour does not affect paramagnetic oxygen analysis.

IX.43 Osmolality:

- A the depression of freezing point of a solution is proportional to its osmolality
- B the water vapour pressure of a solution varies with its osmolality
- C the normal urine osmolality varies from 300–1400 mOsmols/kg
- D a urinary osmolality of 700 corresponds to a specific gravity of 1.040
- E the main determinant of intracellular osmolality is protein.

IX.44 Functional residual capacity:

- A is increased when lying down
- B is 3 litres in a normal young man
- C can be measured by a nitrogen washout technique
- D is increased in pregnancy
- E can be measured by plethysmography.

IX.45 The chi-square test:

- A applies only to continuous variables
- B can prove that one treatment is better than another
- C whether a particular value of chi-square is significant depends on the number of degrees of freedom
- D involves a calculation of expected values
- E can only be applied to normal distributions.

IX.46 Which of the following statements are true:

A the second gas effect explains the actual increase in ventilation due to the rapid entry of nitrous oxide into blood during induction

B the displacement of oxygen from the alveoli by nitrous oxide during recovery from anaesthesia is known as diffusion hypoxia

C for nitrous oxide, an increase in cardiac output will decrease alveolar concentration

D the alveolar concentration of an anaesthetic agent rises more rapidly if ventilation is depressed

E the concentration effect means that inspiration of a high concentration of an anaesthetic will result in more rapid equilibration between alveolar and inspired concentrations.

IX.47 Extracellular fluid:

A contains sodium and chloride as the predominant ions

B has the same osmotic concentration as sea water

C accounts for about 40 per cent of body weight in a normal adult

D includes the plasma volume

E makes a higher proportion of body weight in infancy than in old age.

IX.48 Fluid volumes:

A the normal extracellular fluid volume is 15 litres in a 70 kg man

B total body water is 70% body weight in kilograms

C total body water is simply measured by radioactive labelled chloride ions

D osmolality is the number of osmols/litre

E the normal daily fluid requirement in England is 3 ml/kg/hr.

IX.49 Passage of a current through a wire will depend on:

A the resistance of the wire

B conductivity of the wire

C temperature

D the potential across the wire

E the diameter of the wire.

IX.50 The fidelity of the reading from a trace of direct arterial pressure will be reduced by:

A incompressible fluid filling the system

B gas bubbles

C high compliance of the transducer diapharagm

D a catheter of stiff material

E a long catheter of narrow bore.

IX.51 Diathermy:

    A uses a high frequency current
    B degree of burning depends upon current density at the diathermy tip
    C burns may occur at the earth plate because the same high frequency current flows through the diathermy tip and the earth plate
    D bipolar diathermy coagulation does not require a separate earth electrode
    E if the earth plate becomes detached, the diathermy will not function.

IX.52 Oxygen concentrators:

    A separate nitrogen from the remaining constituents of air
    B utilise a molecular sieve of zeolite
    C are only capable of producing approximately 40% oxygen at a flow rate of 2 L/min
    D depend upon cycling between two separation columns for continuous production of oxygen
    E cycling occurs once every thirty minutes.

IX.53 The pneumotachograph head (Fleisch head):

    A is a method of measuring flow directly
    B integration of the signal gives volume
    C should not be heated to avoid altering the composition of the gas passing through it
    D must be calibrated for a particular gas mixture
    E will only give a linear output over a particular range of flow.

IX.54 Boyle's law:

    A describes the relation between the volume and pressure of a gas
    B is independent of the mass of the gas
    C applies only at constant temperature
    D applies to all gases and vapours
    E is incorporated in the Universal gas law.

IX.55 Possible impurities in commercial nitrous oxide for anaesthetic use are:

    A ammonium nitrate
    B nitric oxide
    C sulphuric acid
    D carbon monoxide
    E nitrogen dioxide.

IX.56 Rotameters:

A   are variable orifice flowmeters
B   the pressure across the bobbin remains constant
C   the increase in area of the annular orifice at high flows reduces resistance
D   in a variable orifice flow meter only laminar flow occurs
E   must be vertical for accurate readings.

IX.57 Pressure:

A   is equal to force divided by area
B   1 Pascal is equal to 102 grams per m^2
C   1000 kPa is equal to 1 Bar
D   1 Bar is the atmospheric pressure at sea level
E   1 Newton is the force which will give a mass of 1 gm an acceleration of 1 metre/sec^2

IX.58 Intraoperative heat loss due to convection is minimised by:

A   increasing the ambient theatre temperature
B   increasing theatre humidity
C   the use of foil wrapping to cover the patient
D   the use of a warming blanket
E   the avoidance of evaporation of spirit based skin preparations.

IX.59 The following are true:

A   logarithms may be to any base, the usual one used is base 2
B 10^{-3} is the reciprocal of 10^3
C   adding the logarithms of numbers is the same as multiplying the original numbers
D   any number raised to the power zero is 1
E   any number raised to the power 1 is the number itself.

IX.60 In acute renal failure:

A   urine output is less than 50 ml/24 hours
B   a blood urea nitrogen to serum creatinine ratio greater than 10 suggests some element of prerenal failure
C   urine osmolarity is less than 100 mOsmols/L
D   in acute tubular necrosis urine sodium concentration is less than 20 mmol/L
E   in acute tubular necrosis urine specific gravity is 1.010 to 1.015.

Paper IX   Answers

IX.1 FTFTT

> **A** There is no such entity as the peripheral nervous system.
> **C** Many other efferents, eg fusimotor fibres, etc.

IX.2 FTFTF

> **A** Intake may be 15 mg of which 3–6% will be absorbed.
> **C** Upper small intestine.
> **E** Phosphate balance is linked with calcium, not iron.

IX.3 TFFFF

> **A** By increasing the pressure gradient from the great veins to the thorax.
> **B** Standing REDUCES venous return for hydrostatic reasons, though compensa– tion occurs quickly in normal subjects.
> **C** It will only be unaffected if there is no compensation for the shunt.
> **D** Exercise increases cardiac output so venous return must rise.
> **E** Aldosterone acts indirectly via sodium balance and ECF volume.

IX.4 FFFTT

Questions about the foetal circulation are asked frequently. You should be able to draw a diagram of the salient features without hesitation.

IX.5 FFFTT

> **A** A-alpha 70–120 m/sec.
> **B** See the explanation to VIII.9
> **C** Peripheral motor portions are usually myelinated.
> **E** True – the amount of acetylcholine released is inversely proportional to the magnesium concentration at the end plate, but that is not nerve conduction.

IX.6   TTFFT

B,C   May produce some difficulty with voluntary movement, but NOT due to intellectual impairment

D   Incoordination yes, but not made worse by closing the eyes, unlike tabes.

IX.7   FFTFT

A   Aldosterone is formed in the zona glomerulosa.

B   It can be difficult to remember exactly figures like the half-life of hormones; what is important is to have some idea of the order of things – ie very short (adrenaline), short (insulin), long (aldosterone) etc.

C   Distal convoluted tubule and collecting duct.

D   Aldosterone increases sodium and water retention, so plasma concen– tration of angiotensin II is decreased.

IX.8   FTTTT

A   Alanine is a product of its synthesis from tyrosine.

B   Yes: 300 times more active than the D-forms.

D   12% to albumin, 88% to thyroxine-binding globulin.

IX.9   FTTFT

A   A rise in systemic blood pressure will be reflected by a rise in intra– ocular pressure but it is not exact and will be modified by local homeostatic mechanisms.

C   Probably true, at least initially, because hypocapnia causes vasoconstriction. Excessive hyperventilation might, however, increase intra– ocular pressure by raising the venous pressure.

D   Glaucoma is more likely if the angle is narrow, but the pressure goes up because of blockage of the canal of Schlemm.

IX.10   FFFFF

Think what one needs to replace after gastrectomy.

B   It is vitamin B12, not intrinsic factor, that is essential and is given as replacement therapy after gastrectomy.

C   It is actually pepsinogen that is secreted, but it isn't essential.

D   Rennin is probably not produced in humans after infancy.

IX.11 TTTTT

IX.12 TTTTF
- **A** All reactions are more likely in atopic individuals, irrespective of prior exposure.
- **E** This may cause hypotension, but not due to hypersensitivity.

IX.13 TFFTT
- **B** Some authorities hold that the pH is the same in the steady-state, others that it is more acid (pH=7.33 compared to 7.40): it is not more alkaline. Buffering and the inter-relations of the acid-base balance of plasma and CSF is a complex subject.
- **C** 75 ml is in the spinal space. Questions that ask if a figure is correct must give a value well outside the normal range for it to be wrong.

IX.14 FTFTF

Mild impairment of glomerular function can be taken as a GFR of 20 to 50 ml/min (a serum creatinine of about 150 to 300 micromol/L).
- **A** Bicarbonate is synthesised in the tubular cells.
- **C,E** Not with mildly impaired GLOMERULAR function.

IX.15 TTTTT
- **B** The central chemoreceptors play no part in hypoxic drive. They are depressed in extreme hypoxia, like most other CNS mechanisms.
- **E** The receptors are thought to be a little way beneath the surface.

IX.16 TFTFT

By definition this is a low V/Q ratio (c) and is the normal state at the base of the lung.

A,B P_AO_2 will fall and P_ACO_2 will rise.

D This is the blood SUPPLYING the alveoli.

E This is so because of the shape of the oxyhaemoglobin dissociation curve: blood from the well ventilated alveoli is already fully saturated.

IX.17 TFTTT

B Angiotensin I is converted to angiotensin II which is unaffected by passage through the lung.

D Velocity is related not to pressure but to flow and diameter of the vessel.

IX.18 FFTFT

A Must be dead space VENTILATION.

B $P_AO_2 = P_IO_2 - P_ACO_2/RQ$: no mention of ventilation here, though ventilation will affect the P_AO_2 indirectly by altering the P_ACO_2.

D 8 ml/kg is too high, it corresponds to 560 ml for a 70 kg man and that would be a high TIDAL volume. A more realistic figure would be 450 – 500 ml, of which 300 – 350 ml would reach the alveoli (5 ml/kg).

IX.19 TFTFF

B It is a represention of the dissociation of oxyhaemoglobin.

D The myoglobin curve is to the left and is hyperbolic not sigmoid.

E Its sigmoid shape is due to the presence of red cells containing 2,3-DPG.

IX.20 TTFTF

C In severe hepatic disease, albumin may fall to 20–25 gm/L

E LDH is also present in skeletal and heart muscle and in red blood cells and so is relatively insensitive as a specific index of hepatic disease.

IX.21 TTFTT

The Rauwolfia alkaloids are now used rarely for the treatment of hypertension but they are important theoretically because of their interactions at the adrenergic nerve terminal; to understand these interactions helps one under- stand the processes at the terminals.

IX.22 TFTTF

B,E   Beta stimulants.

IX.23 FTTFF

There are many thiazide diuretics but none has any advantage over bendro– fluazide, except that chlorthalidone has a longer duration of action and allows prescription on alternate days.

A   Beware the word "mild": don't be tempted to answer unless you know.

IX.24 TFFTT

B   Not documented.
C   Careful! Alterations in serum potassium affect digitalis therapy, but if anything the improvement in renal blood flow would increase potassium loss.

IX.25 FTTTF

A   Calcium, not sodium heparin.
C   Testosterone derivative; plasminogen activator.
D   Snake venom; prevents polymerisation of fibrin leading to the formation of a stable clot.
E   Plasminogen activator used to stimulate fibrinolysis in established clot.

IX.26 TFTTT

    B   They cause relative loss of chloride, hence a hypochloraemic alkalosis.

    C   The major factor in the anti-hypertensive action is probably via a reduction in blood volume.

    D   Look back to IX.23(C): did you give the same answer?

IX.27 FTFTT

Naloxone is a specific opiate antagonist, though there are reports appearing that suggest that, in very large doses, it may reverse the effects of some other centrally depressant drugs.

IX.28 FTTTT

    C   Combined therapy used to be recommended but the incidence of side-effects is too high.

    D   They reduce carbohydrate absorption from the gut and aid peripheral utilisation of glucose.

    E   More likelihood of lactic acidosis.

IX.29 FTFTF

    A,B   It is metabolised, but the rapid initial recovery is because of redistribution to muscle; redistribution to fat is a slower process.

    D   A thiopentone infusion will not give a rapid recovery.

IX.30 TFTTT

    A   Meyer-Overton.

    B   Related to all anaesthetics.

    D   True, Ferguson (1939).

IX.31 TFTFF
- **B**   SVP of ether is 442 mm Hg at 20°C.
- **C**   Increased sympathtic preponderance.
- **D**   No: in fact adrenaline is released during ether anaesthesia.
- **E**   All anaesthetic agents cross the placental barrier readily.

IX.32 TTTFF
- **A**   Liver metabolism: 1% per hour.
- **B**   As are all volatile agents.
- **D**   Destroyed by plasma esterases and then excreted in the urine.
- **E**   Renal excretion.

IX.33 TTFTT
- **C**   Tachycardia secondary to alpha adrenergic blockade.
- **D**   True, although no intrinsic neuromuscular blocking action has been demonstrated.
- **E**   Secondary to atropine-like effect.

IX.34 FTFFF
- **A,C,D,E**   Tinnitus is not associated with any of these drugs although one might expect it to be. Do not guess at an answer of "yes" just because it sounds likely.

IX.35 TFTTT
- **B**   Does not specifically depress respiration even in excess.

IX.36 TFTTT

A   The increase in pressure is not sustained

B   Solutions deteriorate in hot environments and are best kept in a refrigerator, but the answer here is "false".

C   To "should NOT be used" the answer is "true". "Should NEVER be used" could generate much discussion.

IX.37 TFTFF

B   Minimal histamine release.

D   Totally metabolised in plasma.

E   Only mild cardiovascular depression and minimal histamine release, therefore not much vasodilation.

IX.38 TTTTT

IX.39 FFTTT

A,C,D   At the usual dilutions thiopentone (2.5%) is more likely to cause thrombophlebitis than methohexitone (1%). The incidence with propranidid is about twice that with thiopentone.

E   A steroid anaesthetic, a forerunner of althesin. One of the reasons it was abandoned was an unacceptably high incidence of thrombophlebitis.

IX.40 TTTTF

A   Noradrenaline depletion.

B   Renin release leading to rebound hypertension.

C   Altered noradrenaline uptake.

D   Direct acting vasodilator.

E   Probably not because the alpha blocking effect is virtually non-existent.

IX.41 TTFTF

    C   It is designed for this purpose.
    E   Accuracy is dependent upon both viscosity and density because accuracy depends upon laminar flow.

IX.42 TFTTF

    B   Nitrogen is present in the dumb-bell, oxygen in the chamber surrounding them.
    E   Water vapour does affect readings.

IX.43 TTTFF

    D   Corresponds to 1.020.
    E   No – potassium.

IX.44 FFTFT

    A,D It is decreased when lying down or in pregnancy.
    B   It is just over 2 litres in a normal subject, though that depends on sex and height.

IX.45 FFTTF

    A   It applies to occurrences, though they may be of continuous variables – eg the blood pressure being above a certain value in a comparison of different conditions.
    B   Statistics cannot do this. Read about it.
    C   Have a look at a table of the chi-squared distribution.
    E   There are tests (eg the 't' test) that strictly should only be applied to a normal distribution.

IX.46 TTTFT
C   Although only during induction, and relatively less than for a more soluble agent.
D   No, less rapidly.

IX.47 TFFTT
B   Although the ECF is sometimes spoken of as the "internal sea", sea-water is actually hypertonic.
C   20% in a normal adult.

IX.48 TTFFF
C   Deuterium or tritium.
D   MilliOsmols/kg.
E   1–2ml/kg/hr.

IX.49 TTTTT
A,B   Conductivity is the reciprocal of resistance.
C   Strictly yes, although it is only important in thermocouples etc: usually it is the current that produces the temperature

IX.50 FTTFT
Note the wording: "reduced by...". "Fidelity" implies not just accuracy of systolic and diastolic pressures but in the shape of the waveform as well. You must know about natural frequency, damping and critical damping.

IX.51 TTTTF

    C   There must be no high spots or creases in the plate.

    E   The diathermy will function. It will earth by the nearest available route and may cause burns. Most machines have circuitry to detect this type of fault.

IX.52 TTFTF

    A,B   True, zeolite actually traps nitrogen. Oxygen, together with inert gases, passes through the column. On depressurisation, every 45 seconds approximately, nitrogen is "dumped."

    C   Will produce 85–90% oxygen at this flow rate, though maximum rate is about 4 L/min

    E   No – every 30 to 45 seconds.

IX.53 FTFTT

    A   It measures nothing directly, but generates a pressure drop that can be measured by manometers and the flow inferred.

    B   Flow with time = $L\ \sec^{-1} \times \sec = L$.

    C   Heating prevents condensation of water in the fine tubes. Thermostatic control ensures the temperature, and therefore the viscosity, remains constant.

    D   Because of differing viscosities.

    E   A particular head will be calibrated for a range of flow.

IX.54 TFTFT

    B   It is for a given mass of gas.

    D   Strictly it applies only to ideal gases; practically it applies to gases unless close to liquefying. There is no rigid difference between a gas and a vapour: a vapour above its critical temperature is a gas.

IX.55 FTFFT

Hopefully there aren't any!

    A   Nitrous oxide can be manufactured by heating ammonium nitrate, but it is a solid and will not be found as a contaminant.

IX.56 TTTFT

B   True, because it gives rise to a force which balances the force of gravity on the bobbin.
D   Turbulent flow also occurs.
E   There are inclined plane flowmeters, but a Rotameter must be read vertically.

IX.57 TTFTF

B   True, but beware of Pascals not kiloPascals.
C   100, not 1000 kPa (in fact, 101.315 kPa, but 100 is near enough).
E   1 Kg, not 1 gm.

IX.58 TFFFF

B,E   These will only reduce heat loss due to evaporation.
C   Will reduce radiation losses.
D   May prevent some conduction loss, relatively unimportant, but also acts as a heat source.

IX.59 FTTTT

A   The usual bases are e (so-called natural logarithms) and 10.

IX.60 FTFFT

A   Depends upon what phase of renal failure; less than 50 ml/24 hours is anuria, but many patients are only oliguric while many more are in the polyuric phase.
C   Depends upon whether it is due to acute tubular necrosis or prerenal causes, but in neither case does urine osmolarity normally get as low as this – <350 in acute renal failure and >500 in prerenal failure.
D   No – urine sodium is usually greater than 40 mmol/L.

Paper X Questions

X.1 **Double autonomic innervation, from both sympathetic and parasympathetic systems, is not present in:**
- **A** the heart
- **B** the bladder
- **C** the stomach
- **D** the intestine
- **E** peripheral blood vessels.

X.2 **In the metabolism of carbohydrates:**
- **A** glucose is converted to pyruvate by glucose-6-phosphatase
- **B** 5% of ingested glucose will be converted rapidly to liver glycogen
- **C** the rate of entry of glucose to muscle is rate-limiting
- **D** fat is an important input to energy release from carbohydrate
- **E** glucagon raises blood glucose via an effect on liver phosphorylase.

X.3 **Blood volume:**
- **A** is partly regulated by erythropoietin
- **B** influences right and left atrial pressures directly
- **C** is increased by salt loading
- **D** can be measured by a dilution technique using labelled red cells
- **E** returns to normal within 24 hours of a loss of 20% of the initial volume.

X.4 **The cardiac output in a normal adult:**
- **A** rises if the CVP increases
- **B** falls on standing from a supine position
- **C** rises on ascent to 5000 metres
- **D** falls if there is a rise in blood pressure
- **E** falls with an increase in temperature.

X.5 **All-or-none behaviour in relation to nerve conduction means that:**
- **A** a tissue responds to a stimulus if it is large enough
- **B** the size of the propagated action potential is independent of the size of the stimulus
- **C** unless all the synaptic receptors are activated, transmission will not occur
- **D** recruitment does not apply
- **E** the refractory period will be artifically extended.

X.6   Damage or removal of the post-central gyrus of the brain produces:

A   contralateral paralysis of voluntary movement
B   ipsilateral rigidity
C   unconciousness
D   epilepsy
E   contralateral incoordination.

X.7   Parathyroid hormone:

A   mobilises calcium from bone and increases tubular reabsorption of phosphate
B   is regulated by a negative feedback by calcium and phosphate
C   is a polypeptide
D   is regulated by calmodulin
E   is secreted by the chief cells.

X.8   Antidiuretic hormone:

A   release is stimulated by pain
B   release is reduced under halothane anaesthesia
C   release is stimulated by alcohol
D   release can be prevented by regional anaesthesia to L1
E   is available in a synthetic form.

X.9   In the neonate:

A   the tidal volume is 17 ml.
B   the mean blood pressure is 65 mm Hg
C   the haemoglobin is 22–25 G/dl
D   the PaO_2 is a little higher than in the adult
E   the PaO_2 in the umbilical artery will be lower than in the retinal artery.

X.10   In the stomach:

A   there is approximately 8 litres of gastric secretion per day
B   intrinsic factor is secreted by the parietal cells
C   the rate of emptying is slowest after ingestion of fats
D   catecholamines inhibit secretion
E   there is a sterile environment.

X.11 **Fibrinolysis:**
- A is triggered by plasminogen activation
- B interacts with the complement pathway
- C is only activated when bleeding and subsequent coagulation have occurred
- D is unaffected by anaesthesia
- E results in the formation of substances with their own inherent anticoagulent properties.

X.12 **The withdrawal reflex:**
- A is a polysynaptic reflex
- B can be demonstrated by stretching a muscle beyond the length at which the stretch reflex is exhibited
- C as the stimulus increases more limbs will be involved in the response
- D will be faster if the higher centres are intact
- E is an example of a mass reflex.

X.13 **Visceral pain afferents and organs:**
- A the heart and aorta via C5 to T2
- B the adrenals via L1 to L2
- C the uterus via T11 to L2
- D the urinary bladder via T8 to T11
- E the gall bladder via T4 to T10.

X.14 **Renal blood flow:**
- A is approximately 20% of the cardiac output at rest
- B renal cortical blood flow is 12 ml/gm tissue/min
- C medullary blood flow is less than 2 ml/gm tissue /min
- D renal blood flow is measured by inulin clearance
- E effective renal plasma flow is approximately 650 ml/min.

X.15 **There are peripheral chemoreceptors:**
- A situated in the carotid bodies
- B supplied by the glossopharyngeal nerve
- C situated in the adrenal medulla (chromaffin cells)
- D in the aortic arch
- E in the right atrium.

X.16   In a fit, healthy subject breathing 100% oxygen:

A P_AO_2 = 90 kPa (675 mm Hg)
B PaO_2 = 85 kPa (637 mm Hg)
C CaO_2 = 20 ml per 100 ml
D PvO_2 = 7 kPa (52 mm Hg)
E   raising the ambient pressure does not increase saturation.

X.17   On hyperventilating to twice the minute volume:

A   the pH of the blood falls
B   the cardiac output rises
C   the ionised calcium in the blood falls
D   the intrathoracic pressure rises
E   the compliance of the lungs increases.

X.18   One or other form of hypoxia:

A   can be defined as a decrease in blood oxygen tension
B   can be a decrease of oxygen tension in the tissues despite
     normal oxygenation
C   can be an inability of the tissues to use available oxygen
D   can occur despite a normal PaO_2 and peripheral delivery and
     use
E   is exacerbated by hypercarbia.

**X.19   The sigmoid shape of the oxyhaemoglobin dissociation curve of
mammalian whole blood and at 37° C:**

A   facilitates tissue oxygen delivery
B   facilitates oxygen uptake in the lungs
C   is due to the way in which haemoglobin combines with
     oxygen
D   is influenced by the presence of methaemoglobin
E   is independent of venous pH.

X.20   Sodium balance:

A   normal daily sodium requirement is 70–140 mmol
B   normal sodium intake is 10–15 gm/day
C   the sodium content of N/5 saline in 4% dextrose is 20
     mmol/L
D   total exchangeable sodium is more than 90% of total body
     sodium
E   resting intracellular sodium concentration is 5–10 mmol/L.

X.21   Glycopyrrolate:

   A   reduces the tone of the cardiac sphincter
   B   is a more potent drying agent than atropine
   C   is an effective anti-emetic
   D   causes as much tachycardia as hyoscine
   E   can be mixed in a syringe with neostigmine.

X.22   Side effects of ganglion blocking drugs include:

   A   ileus
   B   atony of the bladder
   C   postural hypotension
   D   miosis
   E   bradycardia.

X.23   Glyceryl trinitrate is an effective treatment for angina because it:

   A   raises the threshold of cardiac pain receptors
   B   causes a reflex bradycardia
   C   dilates the coronary arteries
   D   decreases afterload
   E   decreases the blood volume.

X.24   Ouabain:

   A   is strophanthin-G, a cardiac glycoside
   B   the intravenous dose is 2.5 mg
   C   should not be given concurrently with calcium
   D   may precipitate toxicity in a digitalised patient
   E   is not absorbed orally.

X.25   Arvin ("Ancrod"):

   A   is used to lyse established thrombus
   B   prevents polymerisation of fibrin
   C   can cause intraoperative bleeding
   D   is contraindicated in patients with sickle cell disease
   E   is unsuitable for prophylaxis against deep venous thrombosis.

X.26   Hypokalaemia is not a risk with:

A   ethacrynic acid
B   acetazolamide
C   triamterene
D   diazoxide
E   frusemide.

X.27   Metoclopramide:

A   decreases intragastric pressure
B   decreases the gastric emptying time
C   has an action on H2 receptors
D   has an action on the chemoreceptor trigger zone
E   is partially antagonised by atropine.

X.28   The following are true:

A   hydrocortisone replacement alone is sufficient in Addison's disease
B   dexamethasone is suitable for replacement therapy
C   methylprednisolone is five times as potent an anti-inflammatory agent as hydrocortisone
D   prolonged steroid therapy may cause osteoporosis
E   cortisone does not cause fluid retention.

X.29   Ketamine hydrochloride:

A   is related to phencyclidine
B   is available in aqueous solution
C   undergoes N-demethylation
D   the intramuscular dose may be up to 13 mg/kg
E   emergence phenomena are not a problem if used intravenously.

X.30   Etomidate:

A   is an imidazole derivative
B   produces pain on injection
C   maintains cardiovascular stability
D   pharyngeal reflexes are preserved
E   metabolism is first pass dependant.

X.31   Ether:
  A   induced respiratory depression is not associated with severe cardiac depression
  B   depresses bile secretion
  C   produces a rise is CSF pressure
  D   "ether convulsions" are a clinical entity
  E   blood gas partition coefficient is 21.0.

X.32   The following apply:
  A   reducing the dose of phenobarbitone may increase the effect of a dose of phenytoin
  B   potassium potentiates the action qf digitalis
  C   the dose of tolbutamide should be decreased when given with coumarin anticoagulants
  D   ecothiopate eye drops potentiate the action of curare
  E   naloxone increases the respiratory depression of phenoperidine.

X.33   Effects of chlorpromazine include:
  A   alpha adrenergic blockade
  B   antihistaminic action
  C   hypothermia
  D   local analgesia
  E   potentiation of pethidine-induced respiratory depression.

X.34   Tachyphylaxis occurs during treatment with:
  A   ephedrine
  B   trimetaphan
  C   suxamethonium
  D   noradrenaline
  E   sodium nitroprusside.

X.35   Absorption of local anaesthetics from tissues depends upon:
  A   tissue solubility of the agent
  B   vascularity of the tissue
  C   concentration of the drug
  D   rate of breakdown by tissue esterases
  E   local pH.

X.36   Acetylcholinesterase:

A   is found in plasma
B   is inhibited by pilocarpine
C   will hydrolyse dibucaine
D   is present in high concentrations in the placenta
E   hydrolyses acetylcholine faster than other choline esters.

X.37   Vecuronium:

A   is irreversible within 40 minutes of administration
B   is contraindicated in hepatic failure
C   may produce severe hypotension
D   is associated with histamine mediated bronchospasm
E   is metabolised by pseudocholinesterase.

X.38   Pentazocine:

A   has a shorter duration of action than morphine
B   is antagonised by narcotic analgesics
C   is a respiratory stimulant
D   may induce confusion in the elderly
E   is effective epidurally.

X.39   In digoxin overdose:

A   coupled ventricular beats are common
B   overdose is heralded by anorexia
C   toxicity is increased by hypokalaemia
D   toxicity is increased by hypocalcaemia
E   arrhythmias can be treated with propranolol.

X.40   If pethidine is given to a patient receiving monoamine oxidase therapy the following are not unlikely:

A   hypotension
B   ocular palsies
C   coma
D   Cheyne-Stokes respiration
E   cerebral excitation.

X.41   In the electromagnetic flowmeter:

A   blood flow generates a potential by moving through an electric field

B   two probes are used, one which contains the magnetic field coils and another downstream which measures the potential induced

C   depends on blood being a good conductor of electricity

D   the use of an alternating magnetic field improves the stability of measurement

E   the probe only measures the peak flow at the centre of the blood vessel concerned.

X.42   Carbon dioxide analysis:

A   is satisfactorily performed on humidified gas samples using selective infra-red absorption

B   is affected by the presence of nitrous oxide

C   glass is used in the absorption chamber because it does not absorb infra-red light

D   continuous analysis is possible by the infra-red method

E   may be performed chemically using absorption with potassium hydroxide.

X.43   Flame photometry is used to measure:

A   urinary sodium

B   serum potassium

C   serum calcium

D   serum lithium

E   serum magnesium.

X.44   A pressure volume loop will measure:

A   lung compliance

B   airway resistance

C   vital capacity

D   functional residual capacity

E   closing volume.

X.45   For a population sample that shows a normal distribution:

A   the arithmetic and geometric means will be the same

B   96% of the observations will be within two standard deviations of the mean

C   as many values are above the mean as below it

D   there will be no skewness

E   the variance is a function of the mean.

X.46 **Uptake of inhalational anaesthetic agents from the alveoli into the blood depends upon:**

   A alveolar concentration of the agent
   B blood solubility of the agent
   C cardiac output
   D body temperature
   E ventilation/perfusion ratio.

X.47 **The following will distribute uniformly throughout the body water:**

   A urea
   B inulin
   C potassium
   D deuterium oxide
   E Evans blue.

X.48 **Tonicity:**

   A 1 mol of an ideal solute depresses the freezing point by 1.56 deg C
   B tonicity is the effective osmotic pressure in relation to plasma
   C normal plasma osmolarity is 290 mosmol/L
   D the effective osmotic pressure of 5% dextrose is 410 mosmol/L
   E isotonic solutions are non-irritant.

X.49 **The process of diffusion:**

   A the rate depends on concentration gradients
   B of a gas is inversely proportional to the square root of the molecular weight
   C is tested for the lung with carbon monoxide because its diffusion is more rapid than oxygen
   D is unaffected by solubility
   E Graham's law can be applied loosely to liquids.

X.50 **The following are true:**

   A the standard calibration on an ECG monitor is 1 mV=1 cm on the screen
   B the frequency of A.C. in the UK is 60 Hertz
   C a current of 100 milliamps is only just perceptible
   D Ohm's law states that current flowing in a circuit is directly proportional to the voltage and inversely to the resistance
   E the normal voltage of the EEG signal is three orders of magnitude smaller than the ECG.

X.51 The choice of a system for measuring pressure in a blood vessel will depend on:

    A the pressure range
    B the fidelity required in the waveform
    C the availability of apparatus
    D anaemia
    E systemic hypertension.

X.52 Defibrillator:

    A at its maximum setting a potential of 8000 volts is applied across the capacitor plates
    B energy stored is dependent upon charge and potential applied
    C if 400 joules are released the current pulse will be of the order of 35 amperes for 3 msecs
    D the energy required for internal defibrillation is approximately 100 joules
    E when synchronised defibrillation is used, the energy is discharged synchronously with the P wave of the ECG.

X.53 The resistance to flow through a tube:

    A will increase eight times if the radius of the tube is halved
    B is directly proportional to the viscosity
    C is inversely proportional to the length
    D will double if the density of the liquid is doubled
    E can be summarised by the law of Laplace.

X.54 Consider a constant flow of gas along a tube:

    A in total flow energy, the potential energy is reflected by the pressure, the kinetic energy by the velocity
    B beyond a narrowing in the tube the pressure will fall because of the resistance at the constriction
    C the Venturi effect depends on the Bernoulli principle
    D turbulent flow has a flat velocity profile
    E the flow through an orifice placed within the tube may be limited if the pressure drop is high.

X.55 Entonox:

    A is supplied in a cylinder with a shoulder painted blue and white
    B has the same saturated vapour pressure as nitrous oxide at a given temperature
    C may not supply a 50% mixture at low temperatures
    D is commonly supplied via a demand valve in obstetric practice
    E cannot be delivered by a pipeline.

X.56 The critical temperature:

    A for nitrous oxide is 36.5°C
    B is that temperature above which a vapour compressed in a cylinder becomes dangerous to handle
    C is that temperature above which a substance cannot be humidified
    D is used to calculate the filling ratio of nitrous oxide cylinders
    E applies only to vapours.

X.57   Rotameters:

A   density and viscosity of the gas are both important in calibration

B   at low flows, laminar flow occurs and the viscosity of the gas is the most important determinant of flow

C   at high flows the area around the bobbin resembles an annular orifice and gas density becomes important

D   the build-up of electrostatic charge leading to sticking of the bobbin is most likely to occur at the top of the tube

E   bobbins can be interchanged between flowmeter tubes provided that the gas flow rate does not change.

X.58   Solubility:

A   Henry's law states that the amount of a given gas dissolved in a given liquid is directly proportional to the partial pressure of the gas in equilibrium with the liquid

B   as a liquid is warmed less gas is dissolved in it

C   the solubility of a gas depends only upon the gas itself, the temperature, the liquid concerned and the partial pressure

D   the Bunsen solubility coefficient is the volume of gas, corrected to STP, which dissolves in one unit volume of the liquid concerned

E   the Ostwald solubility coefficient is the volume of gas which dissolves in one unit volume of the liquid at the temperature concerned.

X.59   Pressure/force relationship:

A   for a given force applied to a syringe, doubling the diameter of the syringe will reduce the pressure generated by a factor of four

B   the pressure required to open an expiratory valve at its minimum setting is approximately 1.5 cm H_2O

C   the pressure of a full oxygen cylinder is approximately 138 atmospheres

D   Entonox requires only a single stage reducing valve

E   gauge pressure is equivalent to the measured value plus the atmospheric pressure.

X.60   Latent heat:

A   the latent heat of water is higher at 37°C than at 100°C

B   the latent heat of vaporisation of nitrous oxide is zero at 36.5°C

C   at boiling point the latent heat of vaporisation of a liquid is greater than that at its critical temperature

D   if the flow rate of gas from a nitrous oxide cylinder is fast enough to produce icing, the pressure gauge will give a low reading

E   in the respiratory tract, the heat lost in humidifying air is much less than that lost in warming cold air to body temperature.

Paper X Answers

X.1 **FFFFT**

    A,B,C,D,E   Self explanatory: don't get caught out by the negative "not".

X.2 **FTFFT**

    A   Pyruvate is an important compound in intermediary metabolism but is a number of steps from glucose. Glucose-6-phosphatase is an enzyme found in liver and kidney that converts G-6-P to glucose.

    C   Not if insulin is present.

    D   Glucose can be converted to fats via pyruvate and acetyl-CoA, but this reaction is irreversible and there is little conversion of fat back to glucose.

X.3 **FTTTF**

    A   Erythropoietin affects red cell production and maturation, not blood volume.

    D   Red cells can be labelled with ^{51}Cr. Other techniques use albumin labelled with isotopes of iodine.

    E   It takes 12–72 hours to restore the circulating plasma volume. Initially the tissue fluids that are mobilised are virtually electrolyte solutions, protein replacement takes longer.

X.4 **TTTFF**

It can sometimes be very difficult to give dogmatic true or false answers to questions about a system which is so infinitely variable and to which changes rarely occur in isolation. Sometimes, thinking too hard about these questions can cause one to choose the wrong answer.

    D   This begs the question of what caused the (isolated?) rise in blood pressure in a normal adult. This question is true when thinking of peripheral resistance in a heart-lung preparation, but it is not universally true in the intact human.

X.5 **TTFTF**

    C   Red herring.

    E   No – this occurs when the nerve is depolarised repeatedly in quick succession.

X.6   FFFFT

The post-central gyrus is the main sensory area.
C   Not unless the reticular activating system is also affected.

X.7   FFTFT

A   Parathormone increases plasma calcium: remember plasma phosphate is the inverse to calcium so both these statements cannot be true because they imply that calcium and phosphate increase together.
B   Regulation is by calcium, regulation by phosphate is indirectly via calcium.
D   A regulatory protein of calcium at cellular, not plasma, level.
E   The function of the oxyphil cells is unknown.

X.8   TFFFT

B   Increased under halothane.
C   Reduced, leading to well-known diuresis!
D   It may be attenuated, but abolition needs a block to T4.

X.9   TTFFT

A   17–19 ml
D   80 mm Hg
E   True because of right to left shunts below the outflow to the cerebral circulation: the blood to the brain has the highest PaO_2.

X.10   FTTTT

A   3 L. 8 L is the total gastrointestinal secretion per day.
B   The parietal cells secrete hydrochloric acid and intrinsic factor. The chief, or zymogen, cells secrete pepsinogen.

X.11   TTFFT
    C   Continuously activated in a low key.
    D   Enhanced during anaesthesia, particularly by extradurals.

X.12   TFTFF
    The withdrawal reflex is the motor response to a nociceptive
    stimulus.
    B   This is the inverse stretch reflex, for which the afferent is
          the Golgi tendon organ.
    C   The full reponse is difficult to demonstrate in an intact
          animal but can be seen in the spinal preparation – or in a
          patient with a severe spinal or head injury.
    D   The speed of a polysynaptic reflex can vary (unlike the
          monosynaptic) but this is not true.
    E   The withdrawal reflex can be part of the mass reflex.

X.13   FTTFT
    There is no alternative to just learning a list: some people find
    mnemonics are helpful.
    A   T1-T5
    D   T11-L2

X.14   TFTFT
    B   4–5 ml/gm tissue/min.
    D   Para-aminohippuric acid – has a high extraction ratio,
          being secreted as well as filtered. Inulin is used for
          glomerular filtration rate.

X.15   TTFTF
    C,E   The two sites are adjacent to the aortic arch and in the
           carotid body.

X.16 **TTFTT**
  C   22 vols per cent: don't forget that there are significant amounts of dissolved oxygen in hyperoxia.
  D   The PvO_2 may not even be as high as 7 kPa if the cardiac output falls with the hyperoxia and increases the A-V oxygen difference.
  E   The haemoglobin will already be 100% saturated: don't confuse with CONTENT.

X.17 **FFTFF**
This means spontaneous voluntary hyperventilation, not IPPV.
Hyperventilation reduces $PaCO_2$ so **A** is false and **C** is true.
  B   Hypocapnia reduces cardiac output although there will be increased respiratory work.
  D   Mean intrathoracic pressure will not change. The pressure will, however, be lower (more negative) in inspiration and higher in expiration.
  E   The lungs will contain more air but compliance (volume per pressure) will not be affected.

X.18 **TTTTT**
  A   The definition of hypoxic hypoxia.
  B   Stagnant hypoxia.
  C   Histotoxic hypoxia, eg cyanide poisoning.
  D   Anaemic hypoxia: eg low haemoglobin or carbon monoxide poisoning.
  E   Carbon dioxide aids displacement of oxygen from haemoglobin.

X.19 **TTTTF**
  E   A change in pH shifts the curve in both arterial and venous blood.

X.20 **TTFFT** 84 mmol/L
  C   31 mmol/L. 0.9% saline contains 154 mmol/L.
  D   65–70%

X.21   TTFFT
  B   Glycopyrrolate is 5 times as potent a drying agent as
          atropine.
  D   It causes less tachycardia than atropine or hysocine.

X.22   TTTFF
  D   Mydriasis.
  E   Reflex tachycardia due perhaps to parasympathetic
          blockade or to baroreceptor reflex.

X.23   FFFTF
  B   There will be a reflex tachycardia because of the lowered
          peripheral resistance and blood pressure. However
          cardiac work will be decreased.
  C   It will dilate the coronary arteries in normal subjects but
          not in those with angina.

X.24   TFTTF
  B   The maximum intravenous dose is 0.25 mg.
  E   Is rapidly but unpredictably absorbed from the stomach.

X.25   FTFFF
  A   Will only prevent the formation of established clot.
  C   Does not effect immediate haemostasis.
  D   This is a red herring: sickle cell patients do not have
          problems with blood clotting.
  E   It is indicated for DVT.

X.26   FFTFF

NB. "Not a risk."

A,E   It is a loop diuretic, K^+/Na^+ exchange is not prevented.
B   It is a carbonic anhydrase inhibitor, potassium ions are excreted and H^+ conserved.
D   A thiazide-related vasodilator used in the treatment of hypertensive crises.

X.27   TTFTT

A,B   The effect is local, within the stomach wall, and unaffected by vagotomy.
E   The peripheral action is inhibited by atropine.

X.28   FFTTF

A   Fludrocortisone must be given as well.
B   Dexamethasone has little mineralocorticoid activity. It is used mainly in suppression tests and as a potent anti-inflammatory agent.

X.29   TTTTF

A   Phencyclidine was introduced as an anaesthetic giving profound analgesia but was abandoned because of emergence psychosis.
C   You cannot expect (or be expected) to know the answers to all the options in all the questions in an MCQ paper.
E   The route of administration is irrelevant. Not a problem in children, and premedication with benzodiazepines, hyoscine or a major tranquilliser helps.

X.30   TTTFF

B   Depends on the vehicle, and more so in smaller veins.
C   Certainly when compared with thiopentone.
E   Certainly not totally destroyed on first pass.

X.31   TTTTF
- **D**   True: although classically described when ether is given to a pyrexial, toxic child, premedicated with atropine.
- **E**   Blood/gas partition coefficient is 12.

X.32   TFTFF
- **A**   Because phenobarbitone induces microsomal enzymes and this increases the metabolism of drugs given concurrently.
- **B**   No: hypokalaemia increases the likelihood of digoxin toxicity.
- **C**   Because of displacement from plasma proteins.
- **D**   An anticholinesterase: can prolong the action of suxamethonium.
- **E**   The question says "increases" not "reverses".

X.33   TTTTF
- **D**   Many drugs have local anaesthetic properties without being clinically useful as locla anaesthetics.
- **E**   Chlorpromazine has a naloxone-like action, antagonising respiratory depression.

X.34   TTTTT
- **A,B,D,E**   Tachyphylaxis is a phenomenon that is often associated with pressor or hypotensive drugs.
- **C**   Probably linked with the change from phase 1 to phase 2 block that occurs with repeated doses.

X.35   TTTTT
- **E**   Decreased pH in inflamed tissue slows absorption by increasing ionisation.

X.36   FFFTT

A   At the neuromuscular junction, and in the CNS.
B   Pilocarpine is a cholinomimetic used in glaucoma.
C   The confusion here is that dibucaine (cinchocaine) will inhibit the action of plasma cholinesterase and is used in the diagnosis and differentia– tion of atypical cholinesterase.
E   It is also one of the most efficient enzymes known.

X.37   FFFFF

A   Reversible after 15 – 20 minutes.
B   Can be metabolised or excreted unchanged.
C,D No – only mild histamine release, cardiovascularly stable.
E   Is metabolised mainly in the liver, but there may also be non-enzymatic hydrolysis.

X.38   FFFTF

A   Not dramatically different.
B   It is itself a narcotic antagonist, but is not antagonised by narcotics.
C   Not directly, although it will reverse respiratory depression induced by opiates.
E   No, probably because the appropriate opiate receptors are not present in the substantia gelatinosa.

X.39   TTTFT

A   Just about any dysrhythmia can occur in digoxin toxicity.
B   Anorexia is amongst the earliest evidence of overdose.
C,D No: by hyPERcalcaemia. Potassium and calcium are frequently antagonistic.
E   Phenytoin, lignocaine and potassium are the most effective (BUT don't give potassium if the K^+ was high initially). Quinidine, procainamide and propranolol are sometimes effective but frequently produce new arrhythmias.

X.40   TTTTT

Such responses only occur in about 10% of patients receiving both drugs and are probably because of interference with metabolism. Pethidine overdose causes similar symptoms, with an initial rise and then a fall in blood pressure, etc.

1.41   TTTTF

E   The potential developed is proportional to the average blood flow because the flow across the vessel varies and affects the generated potential.

1.42   TTFTT

A   True, water vapour can be absorbed in the sampling line.

C   Glass does absorb infra-red light. The walls of the chamber are made from sodium chloride or bromide crystal.

1.43   TTFTF

C,E   Flame photometry is used basically for urinary or serum sodium and potassium measurements. Since lithium is used as a standard, it is possible also to measure serum lithium levels in the treatment of depressive illness.

1.44   TFTFF

This is a very similar question to 1.41: see the comments to that question for **A** and **B**.

C   VC can be measured by simple spirometry, but it can be read from a pressure-volume loop.

D,E   No: FRC by plethysmography or dilution technique, CV by inhalation of a marker gas (eg 100% O2). You must know the theory underlying these measurements.

1.45   FTTTT

A   They will not be the same because a geometric mean is calculated by taking logarithms to correct skew.

X.46   TTTTT

X.47   TFFTF
> **A**   Urea is a small, soluble, uncharged molecule.
> **B,D,E** Indicator techniques of measurement of volume rely on the indicator's being ditributed uniformly throughout that compartment: inulin – ECF; deuterium oxide – total body water; Evans blue – plasma volume.
> **C**   Administered potassium will certainly be distributed throughout the body but the question states "uniformly"

X.48   FTTFF
> **A**   1.86°C.
> **D**   5% dextrose is isosmotic but not isotonic, red cells put in it will eventually burst because the dextrose is taken up and metabolised, lowering the osmolarity of the solution Note also that osmotic PRESSURE must be measured in UNITS of pressure.
> **E**   Not necessarily.

X.49   FTFFT
> **A**   Only in a single phase. More universally it is the tension gradient that matters. For charged molecules, the electrochemical gradient is important.
> **B**   Graham's law.
> **C**   True but wrong reason: because haemoglobin has such high affinity for carbon monoxide, the rate of diffusion is independent of pulmonary blood flow.
> **D**   When considering the overall process of diffusion, more soluble agents will diffuse faster.

X.50   TFFTT
> **B**   50 Hz.
> **C**   A current of less than 1 milliamp is perceptible; 100 milliamps is a severe shock that could precipitate ventricular fibrillation.
> **D**   Or: V=IR.
> **E**   An order of magnitude means a power of ten: the ECG is measured in millivolts and the EEG in microvolts, three orders of magnitude.

X.51   TTTFF

  A   For example: a water manometer will give a reading of central venous pressure but is not suitable for arterial pressure.
  D,E The choice of apparatus will not "depend on" these conditions, although it might be better, clinically, to have a direct arterial trace during some operations that one might expect to perform on a hypertensive, eg major vascular surgery.

X.52   TTTFF

  D   Internally, usually 50 joules maximum.
  E   Energy is synchronised with the R wave.

.53   FTFFF

The Hagen-Poiseuille formula summarises laminar flow: you can assume flow through a simple tube is laminar unless otherwise stated. Take care to note whether a question is asking about changes in the FLOW or in the RESISTANCE to the flow.

  A   Radius to the 4th power: therefore 16 times.
  D   Density is a factor in turbulent flow.
  E   Laplace's law governs the pressure within surfaces.

.54   TFTTT

  B   Total energy = PE + KE. Velocity (KE) will increase at a narrowing so pressure (PE) must decrease.
  E   The so-called "critical orifice" can be used in gas mixing devices because the flow through the orifice is dependent only on the diameter of the orifice.

55   TFTTF

  B   Entonox, a mixture of gases, cannot have a saturated vapour pressure.
  C   Below $-5.5°C$ some may condense and the liquid phase will be 80% N_2O + 20% O_2. Initial supply will then be hyperoxic, later supply anoxic.

X.56   TFFFF
The critical temperature is that temperature above which a gas cannot be liquefied no matter what pressure is applied. The critical pressure is the pressure at the critical temperature.
C   Liquefied, not humidified.
B,D The filling ratio is defined for safety and ensures that the pressure in the cylinder can never become dangerously high. Critical temperature does not enter into the calculation: it is "critical" because it describes the physica behaviour of the gas.

X.57   TTTFF
D   More likely at the bottom of the tube where it is narrower.
E   Each tube and bobbin are calibrated together for a specifi gas and would be inaccurate for a gas of different viscosit or density.

X.58   FTTFT
A   Henry's law only applies at a given temperature.
D   Only applies where the partial pressure of the gas above the surface of the liquid is one standard atmosphere.

X.59   TTTFF
D   Two stage valve required.
E   Measured value only.

X.60   TTTTF
B   True, 36.5°C is the critical temperature of nitrous oxide.
D   True, fast gas flow, which produces cooling, lowers the vapour pressure inside the cylinder
E   Much more heat is required to humidify air than to warm it.

Index

Questions are listed under broad headings only. There is some overlap between categories, no question is listed more than once.
Roman numerals indicate the number of the paper, and the arabic number that follows is the number of the question on the paper.

Physiology

Pharmacology